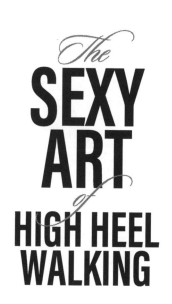

The
SEXY
ART
of
HIGH HEEL
WALKING

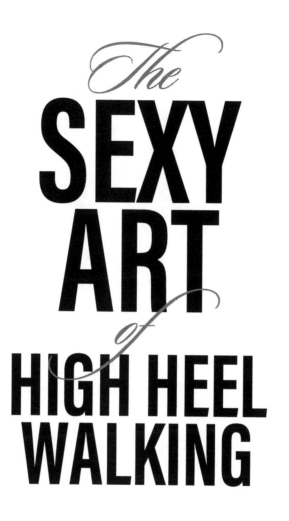

The SEXY ART of HIGH HEEL WALKING

How to Wear High Heels Pain-Free

GIGI SITON, DPT
Doctor of Physical Therapy

THE SEXY ART OF HIGH HEEL WALKING

Printed in the United States of America.

ISBN: 978-0-9991383-0-4

First Printing: July 2017

*This book is lovingly dedicated
to the memories of my amazing parents:
"Papa George" Atty. George L. Siton, Sr.
And
"Mama Lilling" Eligia Flores Siton*

Table of Contents

Acknowledgments

Many people in my life have supported me, believed in me, given me hope, and shared with me information that changed my life. The list is extremely long, and I am limited for space, so thanks to everyone who continues to be a part of my life. You know who you are. Thank you, thank you, Maraming Salamat!

I would also like to thank my beautiful daughters, Alexandra Siton Till and Victoria Siton Till, for being my inspiration in all that I do.

My personal thanks to the excellent Holistic Physical Therapy Team: Mylene Thormer, BSN; Gary Picar, PTA; Minie Puquiz; Annette Norris, LMT; Anekka Roberson; Stevie Dupree, NTP, LMT; Grace Castro, PT; Daniel Lee, LAC; Andrew Magahis, ATC; Tristan Bautista and Alvin Ortiz. Without your unconditional support and commitment day in and day out, Holistic Physical Therapy would not exist. Thanks for helping people every day to regain their health. Most important of all, thanks for believing in and supporting my ideas and vision, and for achieving this company's success at making the world a healthier place in which to live!

I would like to thank Steve and Bill Harrison and the whole Quantum Leap Team for helping my book through the writing, publishing, and marketing stages.

I must thank Emily Ayala and Heidi Grauel, who guided the editing process and held my hand throughout the book writing process. Thanks to Ann McIndoo and Katie Rodgers, my author's coaches, who got this book out of my head and into your hands.

To all my family and friends, too many to mention, thank you for all your support in my personal and professional life.

And, of course, thanks to Pati Bryant of Blossom Photography, an amazing photographer whose photos make me look like a million dollars.

Introduction

Since time immemorial, women young and old have had a fascination with high-heeled shoes. The value of walking in high heels has been ingrained in human consciousness and DNA for all of humanity's four-thousand-plus years' history. High heels project sex appeal, power, grace, and confidence. In this book, I will cover the myths of walking in high heels, the fascinating and juicy history of the evolution of high heels, as well as why high heels are good for you.

As a doctor in physical therapy with almost thirty years of clinical experience, I have extensively studied and applied the biomechanics of walking in all of my patients. In my outpatient holistic physical therapy practice, I see many patients who suffer from foot and ankle injuries. Women with improper footwear and poor high-heeled walking technique will commonly sustain foot injuries. I must admit walking in high-heels is not for everyone. However, for some women who have worn heels for most of their lives, giving up their high heels is like giving up their youth. Eighty percent of women are not confident wearing high-heeled shoes, yet all women would love to learn how to walk in them safely, with grace and confidence.

At my Holistic Physical Therapy Clinic, the final stage of foot and ankle rehabilitation program is the restoration of the patient's static and dynamic standing balance and proprioception sense (how one receives and processes feedback from your body). Mainly, for female patients, I teach unique tips and tools about the sexy art of high heel walking to get them back on their feet safely, with confidence, and pain-free. I have taught everyone from flight attendants and models to prom-going teenagers and women recovering from foot injuries.

There is truly a need to have a book or a formal instruction about the sexy art of walking in high heels. Just as one has to learn how to drive a car before buying one, I believe one should have to learn the sexy art of high heel walking before purchasing high heels. Women, young and old, even men, should be formally taught this sexy art before they purchase high heel shoes, because it is a different skill set from walking in flat shoes.

Amazingly, once you learn all of the principles of the sexy art of high heel walking and proper standing posture, you can apply the same principles—whether barefoot or in whatever shoes you wear—to the rest of your life! Your body will forever thank you for not being tortured in high-heeled shoes. Your feet will be healthy and pain-free ... and, of course, sexy and confident!

Overall, this book focuses on the sexy art of high heel walking without ruining your foot health—it is primarily an injury prevention book. It is my hope that the reader will gain a new appreciation of the historical significance of high-heeled shoes, and learn all of the shoe essentials: shoe anatomy, proper shoe fitting, guidelines for shoe buying, foot health, and appropriate shoe care. Most important of all, you'll learn the correct standing posture and proper high heel walking technique. Wearing high heels can improve posture and balance, and tone the legs, core and pelvic floor muscles. It is like learning how to ride a bike: once you have learned the techniques, you will always know the sexy art of high heel walking pain-free with grace and confidence for the rest of your life!

THE TRUE STORY OF HIGH-HEELED SHOES

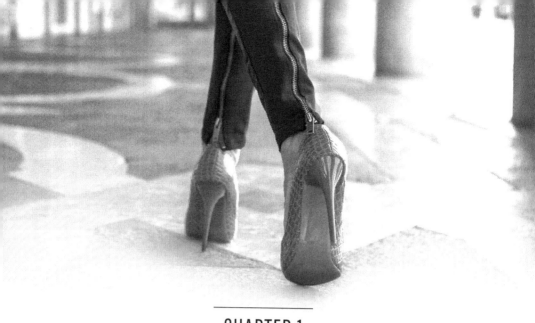

CHAPTER 1

The Origin of High-Heeled Shoes

"Give a girl the right pair of shoes and she can conquer the world."

-MARILYN MONROE

THE HISTORICAL AND SOCIAL CONTEXT OF HIGH HEEL SHOES

For almost four thousand years, the sexy effect of high heel shoes has been ingrained into our subconscious and encoded in our DNA. In ancient Egypt, high-heeled shoes were worn only by the demigods on earth, such as the pharaohs and queens. The shoes were likewise enjoyed by the ancient Greeks and Romans. The French kings' courts used elevated high heels as a fashion statement, although Napoleon outlawed them for a short period of time. They quickly revived back to their original status of boosting one's sex appeal, a revival that has lasted into modern times.

ANCIENT EGYPT

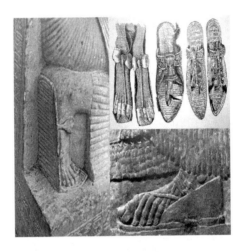

Fig. 1. *Ancient Egyptian heeled shoes[1]*

Let's start tracing the high-heeled shoe from the walls and murals of ancient Egypt. The Pharaohs were determined to maintain their deity status. Wearing sandals or high heels symbolized the separation between the ordinary people (mortals) and the demigods. Pharaohs were considered to be demigods and held absolute power over the masses. Wearing high-heeled shoes projected power and high status. The practical use of high heels is also evident from ancient Egyptian murals, such as those showing butchers walking over animal carcasses in the slaughter house.

ANCIENT ROME, GREECE, AND TURKEY

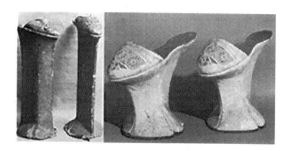

Fig. 2. *Kothorni / Buskins²*

Platform shoes, a type of high-heeled shoes, were used to differenti-ate the social classes between the nobility and the common masses in these ancient cultures. The platform shoes were associated with power: the nobility and dominant ruling classes wore them to save their feet from getting dirty on the dusty Roman streets. They were also used during Roman plays to emphasize the importance of each character.

There was also another significant purpose of high-heeled shoes in ancient Rome: in the legal sex trade they were used to identify a prostitute by potential clients. From then on high heels became asso-ciated with prostitution. From this point in time, high-heeled shoes served not for more practical uses, but gradually became objects of sexual eroticism.

In Turkey, "chopines" were utilized by the nobility to enhance height stature. These were shoes that rose as high as thirty inches and required the aid of two servants just to walk in them. Concubines were made to wear chopines as well, to discourage them from running away from the harem.

EUROPE

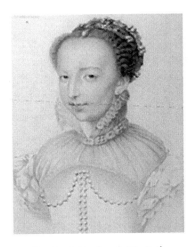

Fig. 3. *Catherine de Medici*[3]

Over time, high-heeled shoes were associated with wealth, power, and nobility. Physical enhancement, particularly increased height, designed to lengthen the legs as a fashion statement, projected authority and status. Catherine de Medici used high heels as a way to compensate for her perceived lack of aesthetic appeal. She felt so insecure with her arranged marriage to King Henry II, knowing that she would be queen of the French Court and in competition with the duke's favorite and significantly taller mistress, the young Diane de Poitiers. Looking for a way to dazzle the French nation and compensate for her looks, Catherine wore two-inch heels, including at her wedding. With the heels she enjoyed a more alluring, towering physique. Before she walked into the French Court, her mother told her to walk slowly and to make each step intentional. Her heels were a wild success. Eventually, the high-heeled shoes grew in popularity and were associated with the privileged class.

Mary Tudor was another royal who pursued heels that would allow her to appear taller than she was. She was determined to wear heels as high as possible to make a grand statement of her power and nobility status. She even wore her high heels when she was walking to her death at the guillotine.

KING LOUIS XIV OF FRANCE

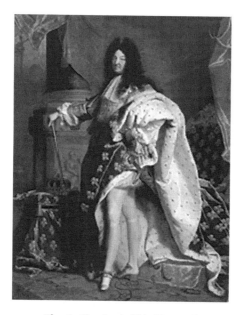

Fig. 4. *King Louis XIV of France* [4]

The Sun King, King Louis XIV, also called "Louis Heels," wore heels as tall as five inches! Fashionable heels were popular for both sexes at the time of the seventeenth century. Louis XIV, a person who had authority and wealth, was often referred to as "well-heeled." The king proclaimed that only aristocrats could wear heels that were colored red, thus, the advent of "red-bottomed shoes." His heels would stack over everyone. He decreed that no one could have heels that were higher than his five-inch heels.

Louis XIV always designed his high heels with miniature battle scenes and elaborate embellishments. When he entered the French Court, his subjects would bow low, enabling them to see his red-bottom shoes with all the decorations on the heels.

MODERN DAY

In the late 1800s, heels were exclusively worn by women and no longer suitable for men. From the end of the 1800s to the 1920s, there were four main types of heels that Western women wore: knock-ons, stacked, spring, and the "Louis".

In the United States, women's fashion gradually improved until in the mid-nineteenth century it caught up with European fashion trends. Cultural influences affected the evolution of the high heel, and it became longer and more slender. High-heeled shoes became associated with the idea of the eroticism of feet and the footwear itself was admired. The use of high heels gave the illusion of aristocracy, associated with wholesomeness, subtleness, and desirability. In contrast, the Puritan British outlawed the use of heels as a way to seduce men.

In the twentieth century, the rise of women's rights had an effect on shoe fashions: the heels stayed under two inches from about 1850 to the 1940s. During the economic crisis of the Great Depression, high-heeled shoes became more practical as a result of the demand for comfortable footwear. Meanwhile, Hollywood introduced a new stylish white and glittery heel, such as those worn by Ginger Rogers. This elegant and flashy style started to challenge the influence of French shoe fashion in the West.[5]

On September 10, 1953, the stiletto was first mentioned in the London's *Daily Telegram*.[6] It was a "Louis" shoe with a narrow heel, stiletto being the Italian word for a small dagger with a slender tapering blade. It came into fashion as a result of collaboration between fashion designer Christian Dior and shoe designer Roger Vivier. Stiletto shoes strongly suggested phallic sexual symbolism. The shoes were very unstable because of the narrow heel design and were banned from public buildings because they caused physical damage to flooring. Their popularity soared when Hollywood starlets Marilyn Monroe and Audrey Hepburn wore them on and off the set in alluring and seductive poses.

Stilettos went out of fashion as the women's liberation movement became popular in the 1960s. The feminist movement associated high heels with women's submission, foot binding, and sexual stereotyping by men.

The 1970s hippie culture was an age of experimentation with drugs, sex, and, of course, fashion. It brought the chunky platform shoe, which was worn by both men and women.

During the 1980s and 90s, high heels continued to evolve and the liberal feminist views of high heels faded. Designers such as Manolo

Blahnik shepherded the return of high heels in these two decades. Resurgence of the popularity of high heels took them from the catwalk to Hollywood and eventually to every woman. The emergence of a new feminist culture associated high heel shoes with feelings of importance, dominance, and authority. Wearing high heels was for a woman's own benefit, not just to be appealing to men.

Chapter Notes

1. Source: nimmafashionsource.blogspot.com
2. Source: nimmafashionsource.blogspot.com
3. Source: madameguillotine.org.uk
4. Source: madameguillotine.org.uk
5. "Dangerous Elegance – A History of high heelShoes." Random History. 2012. Web. 9 November 2012. <http://www.randomhistory.com/1-50/036heels.html>.
6. "Dangerous Elegance – A History of high heelShoes." Random History. 2012. Web. 9 November 2012. <http://www.randomhistory.com/1-50/036heels.html>.

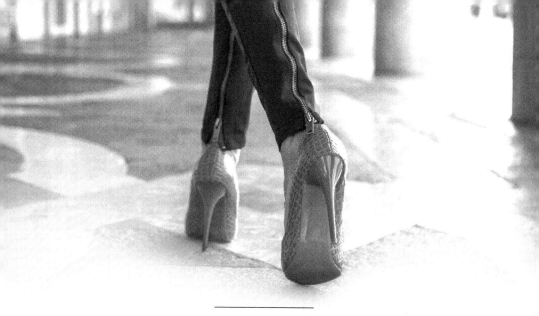

CHAPTER 2

Debunking the Ten Myths of High-Heeled Shoes

"High heels give you time to think, to look at your surroundings—a camel has seen more in life than a very quick horse! Women should live to the rhythm of high heel shoes!"[1]

—CHRISTIAN LOUBOUTIN

Essentially, high-heeled shoes are fashionable although uncomfortable. They are almost exclusively perceived as a threat to foot health and practicality. It doesn't make sense to prefer a type of footwear that could potentially harm and hurt your feet. It may even be a challenge to run from predators in high-heeled shoes. But

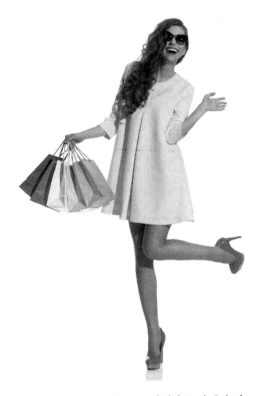

Fig. 5. *Happy Lady on Red High Heels Pain-free*

wearing them makes a woman more attractive and boost her self-confidence, thus enhancing her sex appeal. In short, it is the only fashion statement that has been around for almost four thousand years that gives women evolutionary advantage with both a physiological and a psychological impact on society.

There are two distinct reactions when I ask women their opinions about high-heeled shoe walking. The majority of the younger women seem very excited; in contrast, more mature women have negative views. Occasionally, I encounter very negative responses including blaming high heels for existing bunions or arthritis, or for foot and ankle injuries, or even blaming these shoes for back or neck pain. I would curiously ask these responders if they could tell me what their conceptions about high heels were, and if they ever had proper instruction for walking in high heels. As I suspected, the majority of women were not aware of the sexy art of high heel walking, nor of shoe basics. Most women were sold on the idea of high-heeled shoes, but were not taught the sexy art of high heel walking. The greatest opposition to wearing high heels is the result of poor high heel walking techniques, ill-fitting high heels, and poor standing posture.

The following are ten common myths about wearing high-heeled shoes:

1. HIGH HEELS CAN CAUSE FOOT AND TENDON PAIN.

Foot and ankle sprains and strains are among the most common types of foot injuries. Sprains of the ankle occur when the ankle is accidentally turned or rolled outward or, less commonly, inward. Sometimes ligaments of the ankle are torn, resulting in a lateral or medial sprain. These types of sprains and strains range from first to third-degree injuries.

Foot and ankle sprains and strains could happen whether you are wearing flats, tennis shoes, or even high heels. Such injuries are most likely due to muscle imbalances in foot and ankle, poor balance, poor proprioception, poor shoe fit, poor high heel walking technique, and/or weak core muscles. High-heeled shoes are not the sole reason for foot and ankle sprains and strains. Admittedly, wearing them can aggravate preexisting foot and ankle pain.

2. HIGH-HEELED SHOES INCREASE THE INCIDENCE OF SPRAINS AND FRACTURES.

As I just explained, high heels can aggravate preexisting conditions. The shoes themselves need not be the cause of sprains and fractures. Learning proper balance and technique can help decrease the likelihood of an accident.

3. HIGH-HEELED SHOES MAKE CALVES LOOK MORE RIGID, ALSO CAUSING LOWER LEG AND CORE MUSCLE WEAKNESS.

Proper balance and posture, as utilized in the sexy art of high heel walking, will actually tone your calf muscles, and strengthen core muscles as your body weight is properly distributed and supported. They key is in instructing the wearer with proper form, so that the body is enhanced, not stressed.

4. HIGH HEELS CAN CREATE FOOT DEFORMITIES, INCLUDING HAMMERTOES AND BUNIONS.

When shoe wearing became a necessity and accepted as the social norm, humans developed foot deformities such as hammertoes and bunions. Based on the foot's outstanding design and function, avoiding these deformities depends on proper walking technique and the quality of shoe craftsmanship. Ill-fitting shoes can cause foot pain or many foot deformities such as hammertoe or bunions.

It is convenient to blame high heels as the primary reason for toe deformities. Actually, the majority of patients who suffer foot problems and great toe maladies do not wear high heels. It is true that high-heeled shoes concentrate pressure on the toes, which can aggravate or even cause toe problems, if a person is not aware of the proper high heel walking technique. The sexy art of walking in high heels is a unique skill set. One should receive instruction on this art at least once before walking in high heels. I have worn three- to four-inch high heels all day at work for almost twenty years now, and I don't have foot deformities or any foot pain. This is the reason why I wrote this book. In the coming chapters, I will discuss the basics of proper footwear and the sexy art of high heel walking to prevent foot and toe deformities.

Toe deformities are even evident in men who have never worn high-heeled shoes. The big toe deformities could be due to the malalignment of the whole leg with the core muscles. It is simply the bio kinetics of walking, beginning with the brain, spine, leg, and foot dynamics when the foot hits the ground ... everything changes! It is a complex chain reaction of the gravitational downward pull starting when the foot hits the ground. Then, in nanoseconds, the reaction rebounds back upward to the spine, to the brain, then back to the spine, to the pelvis, to the hip joint, then back down to the legs, to the knees, eventually back to the ankle and all of the toes, especially the big toe. Any weaknesses in any part of the chain reaction at any of these points will ultimately affect the farthest points first: such as the big toes and other neighboring toes, resulting in bunions and hammer toes. Most bunions occur and reoccur, even after surgical repair, if a poor posture and poor walking technique are not corrected.

5. HIGH-HEELED SHOES CAUSE AN UNSTEADY GAIT.

Unsteady gait with high-heeled shoes is the result of poor high heel walking technique or ill-fitting shoes. Wearing high-heeled shoes will elevate your heel higher above the ground while walking. It redistributes the gravitational forces impacting your feet's balance and proprioception sense. During high heel walking, your body's balance is actively challenged, which can result in unsteady walking. Learning the sexy art of walking in high heels with proper fitting shoes will correct unsteady gait.

6. HIGH HEELS SHORTEN THE WEARER'S STRIDE.

The fundamentals of the sexy art of walking in high heels is to take smaller steps. High heel shoes are not meant for big-stride walking but instead for smaller steps, very intentional, mindful ... sexy walking. The sexy art of high heel walking technique is supposed to enhance sex appeal and attractiveness. As designer Christian Louboutin so colorfully stated, wearing high-heeled shoes enables you to slow down and enjoy every step while soaking in your surroundings. It is a form of mindful walking in life.

7. HIGH-HEELED SHOES CAN RENDER THE WEARER UNABLE TO RUN.

High-heeled shoes are NOT for running, which is why they are not the preferred footwear in the gym. If you must run with high heels, carry them in your hand. Then you can run.

8. HIGH-HEELED SHOES CAN EXACERBATE LOWER BACK PAIN.

True, it is not a good idea to wear high heels if you have lingering lower back pain. Poor posture and weak core muscles combined with chronic dehydration are common causes of non-traumatic lower back pain—naturally, high heels just exacerbate the problem. It is important to note that the majority of lower back pain patients are not wearers of high heels. Many men and women have lower back pain, without ever having worn high-heeled shoes.

9. HIGH-HEELED SHOES CAN ALTER FORCES AT THE KNEE SO AS TO PREDISPOSE THE WEARER TO DEGENERATIVE CHANGES IN THE KNEE JOINT.

High-heeled shoes do NOT predispose any individual to degenerative knee disease. Joint degeneration, particularly in the knee joint, is primarily due to poor nutrition, poor lifestyle choices, and weak core and leg muscles. Poor high heel walking technique will increase stress on the preexisting weak knee and poor foot alignment. Eventually, weak leg muscles will weaken knee joints, when one walks on high heels with knees bent. However, with the sexy art of high heel walking, core and leg muscles will grow stronger.

Everyone knows of the legendary Tina Turner's million dollar pair of legs! She has always worn high-heeled shoes for walking or dancing while performing in her concerts for years. It doesn't look like her high-heeled shoes cripple her. I believe that her well-defined leg muscle tone and strength at 77 years old could be the cumulative effect of years of high-heeled shoe walking.

I always suggest to my patients that if they do not have time to work out, the sexy art of high heel walking for an hour a day will challenge their core and leg muscles. And it can improve dynamic standing balance and proprioception to boot. (I'll explain more about these benefits later.)

10. HIGH-HEELED SHOES CAUSE DECREASED ANKLE AND FOOT ROTATION BECAUSE THESE SHOES MAKE THE KNEES WORK HARDER.

It is true that high heel shoe walking will reduce ankle and foot rotation. It does make the knees work harder. However, learning and mastering the sexy art of high heel shoe walking can help with this dilemma. It can be corrected by walking with an increased side hip sway. The knee is locked during heel strike to make up for the decreased ankle and foot rotation. The ankle plantar flexed position in high heels will be offset by the exaggerated hip side sway. Hence the knees will work less and become efficient and, as a result, will be protected. I hope I did not lose you with the technical mumbo jumbo. In short, just stick with the sexy art of high heel walking, and you can minimize the stress to the knees.

Dispelling the ten myths of high-heeled shoes is an important first step to learning the sexy art of high heel walking. This unique skill set will prevent foot injuries and, what is more important, you'll be able to enjoy walking in high heels. You will master the power walk pain-free with grace and confidence.

Chapter Notes

1.   http:/justheels.net/ Just Heels by Zuzana Annal, May 20, 2916

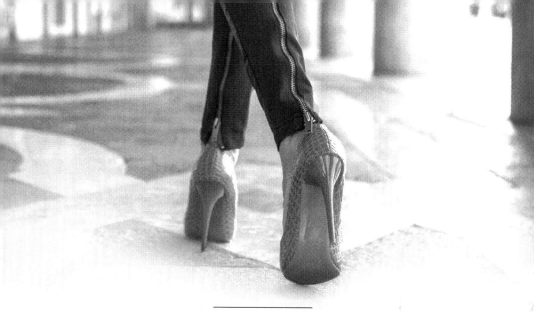

CHAPTER 3

High Heels Are Good for You!

"Shoes transform your body language and attitude.
They lift you physically and emotionally."

—CHRISTIAN LOUBOUTIN

High-heeled shoes are good for you! There are so many benefits to be gained from wearing high-heeled shoes daily or occasionally once you learn the proper technique of the sexy art of high heel walking. Walking in high heels pain-free and effortlessly with grace could be your secret weapon for massive sex appeal and boosted self-confidence. High-heeled shoes are an important fashion essential worn by top power women in fashion, high society, and politics. The right footwear, like high heels, projects your importance in every formal and social occasion including parties, birthdays, homecoming, prom, and, of course, weddings, to name a few.

The following are the eight benefits of high heel walking:

1.   HIGH HEELS ARE GOOD FOR YOUR BRAIN!

We all know that maintaining good upright posture and having good standing balance are important in walking on high heels the proper way. This is the job of the cerebellum which is located at the back of the brain. The cerebellum's main job is to control all movement-related functions. It is responsible for good posture and anything to do with standing balance, also known as equilibrium. It coordinates precision and accurate movement timing. It receives signals from the sensory antennae of the spinal cord, from the trunk, arms, legs, and from other parts of the brain. One's cerebellum integrates these signals for a fine-tune movement such as high heel walking.

High heels encourage the wearer's posture to be more upright in the chest, resulting in a good, upright posture. (You'll learn the complete instruction in Section C: Mastering the Sexy Art of High Heel Walking: Chapters 6, 7, 8.) Standing and walking on high heels will improve your static (stationary) and dynamic (moving) standing balance which will continuously challenge and improve your brain function.

Also, proper high heel walking is a learned skill that will promote neuroplasticity of your brain. Neuroplasticity is the latest development in neuroscience as explained in Dr. Norman Doidge's book:

The Brain That Changes Itself. It means that your brain is plastic and pliable. It will always continue to grow and evolve if you are constantly learning new skills and challenging it every day regardless of your age. Proper Posture + Proper Dynamic Standing Balance while Walking in High Heels = Healthy Brain!

2. HIGH HEELS ARE GOOD FOR INCREASING ONE'S ATTRACTIVENESS FACTOR.

High heels make the feet appear smaller, which increases the attractiveness of feet, or "the Cinderella Effect." Studies have shown that men are attracted to women with smaller feet. A recent paper in the March 2012 issue of *Evolution and Human Behavior* by Dan Fessler et al. investigated aesthetic preferences of feet. Women with smaller feet, but with equal attractiveness, always had the advantage. Fessler and his colleagues conducted a substantial number of follow-up studies, mostly showing similar patterns, with one exception. In an Indonesian population, women with large feet were preferred. This finding seems to imply that multiple factors might influence foot aesthetics, and the economic importance of walking around in this rural population might affect what is seen as attractive.[1]

One study showed men and women experimental stimuli and then asked if they could identify how the images differed from one another. Nearly 40% of male subjects correctly identified feet as the factor that stood out, while less than 20% of the female subjects were able to do so. It appears evident that women do not pay sufficient attention to footwear compared to men on this particular study.

High heel walking encourages a seductive gait to accommodate the shoes when worn correctly. High heel shoes elongate the legs, making the wearer seem taller and increasing sex appeal.

3. HIGH HEELS ARE GOOD FOR ONE'S CORE, PELVIC FLOOR, AND LEG MUSCLES.

High heel walking requires having your core muscles always activated to maintain a proper posture and to lessen the impact on your feet. The core muscles are strengthened by constant isometric activation of the postural abdominal muscles in the front and the spinal muscles in the back, while one is walking on high heels. Thus, wearing high heels strengthens your core, leg, and feet muscles. High-heeled shoes emphasize the calves' appearance due to the change in angle

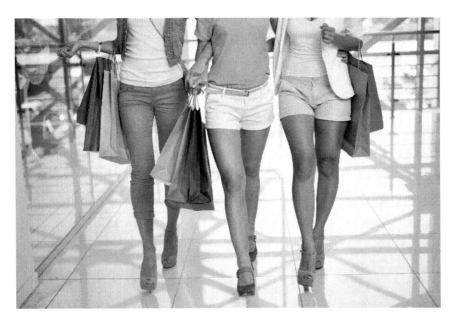

Fig 6. *Strong legs and feet in high heels*

of the feet when pointing downward. They also emphasize the feet's arches, giving better definition and height.

According to a single line of research, high heels may stimulate the muscle tone of the wearer's pelvic floor, thus possibly reducing female bladder incontinence, although these results have been challenged.

I daresay that high heel walking can be a good exercise for strengthening core muscles, pelvic floor muscles, and leg muscles while improving dynamic standing balance.

4. HIGH HEELS ARE GOOD FOR YOUR PSYCHE.

It is a common fact that women have a long history of shoe fascination, even to the point of shoe obsession for some women. Fairy tales such as *Cinderella* and her glass slippers that led to everlasting love with Prince Charming are an example of how young girls are introduced to a love of shoes. Remember Dorothy in *The Wizard of Oz* where the ruby slippers held all the power for her wishes and her ultimate freedom from the Emerald City? How about Imelda Marcos, from my country the Philippines, who was notorious for her massive collection of more than ten thousand pairs of expensive shoes? Or, Carrie Bradshaw of *Sex in the City* and her shoe collection and love affair with her exquisite and expensive shoes?

For centuries, high-heeled shoes have evolved to serve many different purposes: from representing demigods, to the power of eroticism, to female bondage, to a fashion statement for both men and women. Eventually, men stopped wearing high-heeled shoes; however, women's fascination with high heels, clothes, wigs, jewelry, and makeup persists.

In 2007, Consumer Reports National Research Center polled 1,057 women and found that, on average, the women owned 19 pairs of shoes. Although, they wore only four pairs regularly, while 15% had over 30 pairs of shoes. As a matter of fact, I checked my closet, and I found that I have 168 pairs of shoes—half of which are high-heeled shoes. I make it a point to wear each pair of high heels more than once per season ... At least I'm honest!

The same article from Consumer Reports also documented shoe injuries, stating: a total of 43% of women claimed they were moderately injured by shoes, and 8% reported serious injuries from sprains or even fractures. I am curious to know if these injuries could have been prevented if the wearers had been taught the proper technique of high heel walking.

I have two teenage daughters, and they have always been fascinated with my high-heeled shoes. When each of my daughters turned thirteen years old, she, like so many other girls, slipped those ruby reds on her feet and was transformed into a beautiful woman. The shoe industry is well aware of why women love shoes and they capitalize on the fact that they make women feel more beautiful, more attractive, taller, thinner ... Very valuable commodities![2]

5. HIGH HEELS ARE GOOD FOR YOUR CONFIDENCE.

Walking in high heels is the ultimate power walk because it projects internal power with grace and confidence. Once you master the sexy art of high heel walking, you will have the secret to the ultimate power walk. It is a particular skill set of walking that is easier to learn than you think, if it is taught correctly. Heels make the wearer look taller and feel larger than life.

"Well-heeled" is a term that was used for centuries to describe nobility who had wealth and authority. Therefore, high heels even today are associated with high society or high economic status. This psychological impact of high-heeled shoes can be traced historically for four thousand years—a connection that I believe has resulted in encoding their appeal deep in our DNA, consciously and subconsciously.

Good posture on high heels is super sexy. Posture projects power! The proper high-heeled standing pose can help to achieve the ultimate confidence for a power walk. Everyone has heard acclaimed speaker Amy Cuddy's talks on power posing. Cuddy explains that an open, expansive posture reflects high power, while a narrow, closed posture reflects low power. These poses not only show an impression of power, but can actually produce it. An individual with high power poses has boosted feelings of dominance, risk-taking, and power, as well as decreased anxiety.[3] It means that high power poses + high-heeled shoes = massive confidence!

6. HIGH HEELS ARE GOOD FOR YOUR SEX APPEAL.

In modern society, high-heeled shoes are a part of women's fashion, especially as a sexual prop. High-heeled shoes force the body to tilt, emphasizing the buttocks and breasts. They highlight the role of feet in sexuality, and the act of putting on stockings or high heels is often seen as an erotic act. This desire to look sexy and erotic continues to drive women to wear high-heeled shoes, even when it causes significant pain in the ball of the foot, or bunions or corns, or hammertoe. A survey conducted by the American Podiatric Medical Association showed some 42% of women admitted that they would wear a shoe they liked even if it gave them discomfort.[4]

Psychologists Paul Morris, Jenny White, Edward Morrison, and Kayleigh Fisher from the University of Portsmouth, in the UK, have recently proposed a novel evolutionary theory about why women favor high heels. "As women normally walk differently from men, high heels may help exaggerate the particularly feminine aspects of gait. What these shoes do is make women walk even more like women." In their recent study, entitled "High heels as supernormal stimuli: How wearing high heels affects judgements of female attractiveness," the psychologists compared ratings of women walking in flat shoes with the same women walking in high heels, in order to establish whether or not walking in high heels enhances the attractiveness of gait.[5] The study, published in the academic journal *Evolution and Human Behavior*, found that for all walkers, attractiveness was rated much higher in heels compared to flat shoes. Both males and females judged high heels to be more attractive than flat shoes. Men and women also agreed on which walkers were the attractive ones and which were unattractive.

The authors of the study concluded that high heels are an important part of the contemporary female wardrobe—the minimum number of high-heeled shoes owned by those taking part in the experiment was four, and the maximum twenty-five.

The results indicate that the female walk is perceived as much more attractive when wearing high heels than not. One motivation for women to wear high heels, whether conscious or unconscious, therefore, might be to increase their attractiveness.[6]

7. HIGH HEELS ARE GOOD FOR INCREASING MEN'S PROFESSIONAL AND SOCIAL ATTENTION ... AND RESULT IN QUICKER RESPONSE!

In another study completed in 2014, Nicolas Guegeun[7] examined the impact of shoes in four series of experiments. In all of these four experimental scenarios, Gueguen recruited college-aged women dressed in matching outfits—straight black skirt, white long sleeves, and black suit jacket—but with heel height variation. He then engaged the subjects in a series of tasks on the street and measured the reactions of those passing by.

The first two experiments focused on the participants' willingness to comply with a survey request on equal rights and dining preferences presented by an interviewer wearing either heels or flats. The results revealed that interviewers in higher heels received an active compliance response from male participants, ranging from between 82% and 83% eagerness, compared to 42% to 47% when the interviewer was wearing flat shoes. However, the female participants had a lower participation rate, only 30% to 36%, and this was consistent no matter which type of heel was worn by the female surveyor.

The third experiment attempted to measure the effects of high heels on helping behavior of both men and women responders. The same group of female participants, walking in shoes with different heel heights, dropped a glove on the floor and waited to see whether someone noticed and helped them. The results revealed that male participants responded 93% of the time, which was directly related to higher heel height; the helping response was only 62% when the woman was wearing flats. Meanwhile, the shoes had no effect on the female participants' helping behavior—the response rate was consistently 43% to 52%.

In the final experiment, the female participants were dispatched to a bar wearing heels of different heights. The study was designed to measure the amount of time it took for a man to notice and approach a woman, based on the shoes she was wearing. The women who wore higher heels were approached sooner—at eight minutes after entering the bar—compared to fourteen minutes for a woman in flats. Men were more attracted to a lady in high heels. The study affirmed the fact that men perceived women in a higher heel to be more influential and more alluring.

According to Jeremy Nicholson, Ph.D., the persuasive effect on high heels seems to be connected to sex appeal.[8] It significantly influences men and increases attention in a bar—and, men could be more compliant to requests and behave more helpfully. Essentially, wearing high heels could increase a woman's social and professional response from men.

8. HIGH HEELS ARE GOOD FOR FIRST IMPRESSIONS.

Everywhere I go, people always notice my high heels. They have been a good icebreaker to conversation in multiple social situations. A study from the *Journal of Research in Personality*, by researchers from the University of Kansas and Wellesley College, found that certain shoe characteristics are telling of the wearer's personal traits.[9] The subject's gender, age, and income, as well as a few subtle personality traits, were accurately predicted when college students observed photos of other people's favorite shoes. The personality tests taken by the wearers showed the respondents' assumptions were accurate. The study shows that shoes are a helpful tool in forming first impressions.

For Meghan Cleary, who last year published the book *Shoe Are You?*, as an update to her 2005 book, *The Perfect Fit: What Your Shoes Say about You*, the University of Kansas-Wellesley study was a welcomed qualitative affirmation of the power of shoes to express personality.[10] "It's this physiological impact," Cleary said. "Shoes are the only fashion item we put on our bodies that have both a physiological and psychological impact."[11]

Chapter Notes:

1. http://epjournal.net/blog/2012/03/another-cinderella-effect-the-attractiveness-of-feet/ Another Cinderella Effect? The Attractiveness of Feet ...

2. The Psychology of Women–What is the Meaning of High ... https://www.psychologytoday.com/blog/in-the-trenches/200909/the-psychology-women-what-is-the-meaning-high-heels

3. https://www.ted.com/talks/amy_cuddy_your_body_language_shapes_who_you_are

4. What about high heel Shoes?–Truediscipleship. http://truediscipleship.com/what-about-high-heeled-shoes/

5. Why high heels make women more attractive | Psychology Today. https://www.psychologytoday.com/blog/slightly-blighty/201508/why-high-heels-make-women-more-attractive

6. Why high heels make women more attractive by Raj Persaud, MD, and Professor Adrian Furnham, MD. www.psychologytoday.com/blog/slightly-blighty/201508/why-high-heels-make-women-more-attractive

7. Guéguen, N. (2014). High heels increase women's attractiveness. Archives of Sexual Behavior, 1-9.

8. Jeremy Nicholson, MSW, Ph.D.; https://www.psychologytoday.com/blog/the-attraction-doctor/201412/the-surprising-power-women-in-high-heels

9. Shoes as a source of first impressions

10. *Chicago Tribune*; A sling back state of mind June 26, 2012|By Alexia Elejalde-Ruiz, Tribune Newspapers aelejalderuiz@tribune.com

11. Shoe personalities: Study shows you can judge people's http://articles.chicagotribune.com/2012-06-26/features/sc-fash-0625-shoes-personality-20120626_1_shoes-round-toed-personality

SECTION B

CHOOSING THE RIGHT SHOE FOR YOU

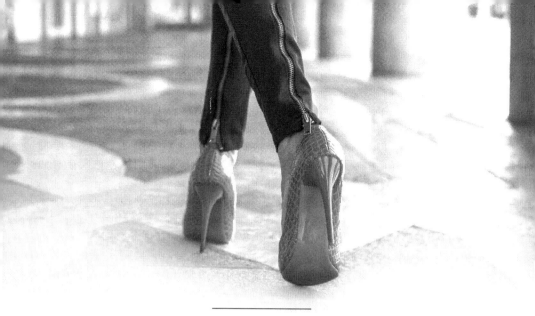

CHAPTER 4

What's Really in a Shoe?

"You put high heels on and you change."

- MANOLO BLAHNIK[1]

FASHIONABLE HIGH HEELS

High heels presumably give the illusion of longer, more slender legs.

There are two heel classification systems:

1. **The shoe industry:** high fashion shoes, such a Jimmy Choo and Gucci, categorize high heels as follows:

- 1- to 2.5-inch heel equals a *low heel*
- 2.5- to 3.5 inches is considered a *mid-heel*
- 3.5 inches or higher is considered a *high heel*

2. **The clothing industry:** perceives anything between 2 inches to 5 inches to be a high heel.

These are the popular and current high-heeled fashion shoe styles:

STILETTO

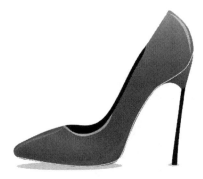

Fig. 7. *Stiletto*

The stiletto is known for its pencil-thin, dagger-like heel, sure to lengthen even the shortest legs. It is still the most popular high-heeled shoe fashion, though it has been around a long time.

PUMPS

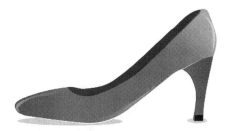

Fig. 8. *Pumps*

Pumps–an attractive high-heeled style for over a century, a classic standard pump heel is a little bit thicker than the stiletto heel.

PEEP-TOE

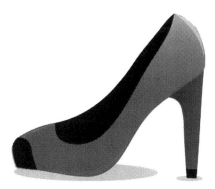

Fig. 9. *Peep-Toe Shoes*

Peep-toe is an innovative combination of a peep-toe and sandal styles to reveal "a little bit of toe."

WEDGE

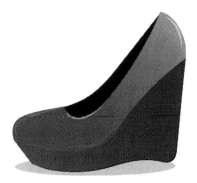

Fig. 10. *Wedge Shoes*

A wedge is a more comfortable casual choice than the stiletto, with a stable heel throughout the length of the foot. It is preferred by many women due to its stability and comfort.

PLATFORM

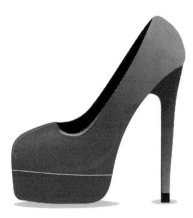

Fig. 11. *Platform High Heel Shoes*

The platform shoe is a 1970s-inspired high heel that enhances all-over height in varying styles such as pumps and wedges.

SANDALS

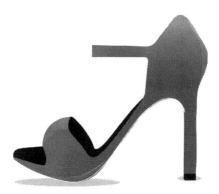

Fig. 12. *High Heel Sandals*

Sandals have an open and casual high-heeled style with ankle straps for a better shoe fit, making them more stable for walking. They are more secure, and allow for comfortable walking and dancing.

KITTEN HEELS

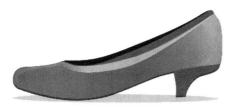

Fig. 13. *Kitten Heels*

Kitten heels have a small hint of a heel but are slenderizing and more comfy for walking.

COWBOY BOOTS

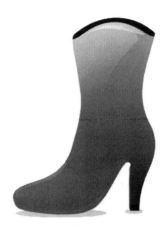

Fig. 14. *Cowboy Boots*

Cowboy boots are a country-inspired look that is rustic and fun, and comes in high heels or flats.

SLING BACKS

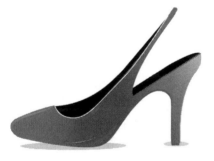

Fig. 15. *Sling backs*

Sling backs are comfy and easy to wear—they just slip on. They offer more security than some other heels, and allow for comfortable walking and dancing.

ANATOMY AND PARTS OF A HIGH-HEELED SHOE

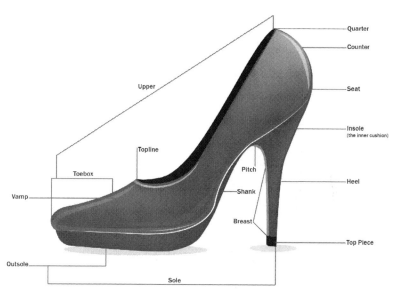

Fig. 16. *Anatomy of a High Heel*

Breast – The forward facing part of the heel, under the arch of the sole.

Counter – A stiff piece of material at the heel of a shoe positioned between the lining and upper that helps maintain the shape of the shoe. The counter helps strengthen the rear of the shoe.

Feather – The part of the shoe where the upper's edge meets the sole.

Heel Height – This can be anywhere from 2 to 6 inches, or higher. Even though the media (and retailers) imply that women only wear stilettos, that is not true. Nor is only wearing stilettos healthy for your feet or back. About 2.5 inches is a good maximum height for heels worn on a daily basis.

Heel – The heel is the part of the sole that lifts the rear of the shoe in relation to the front.

Heel Width – Generally, high heels are thinner, although it is stylish now to wear a chunky platform heel which may be quite high. If you do not like high heels but want the illusion of wearing them, wear kitten heels which are low but thinner and give you the look of wearing heels.

Last – This is a model of the foot that establishes the arch, thereby determining how your weight is distributed along the length of your foot. If your arch does not conform to it, the shoe will always be uncomfortable. This is why it is very important to try on both left and right shoes and walk around in them before purchasing.

Lining – Most shoes include a lining on the inside of the shoe, around the vamp and quarter. A lining improves comfort and can help increase the lifespan of the shoe.

Outsole – The exposed part of the sole that is in contact with the ground. As with all parts of the shoe, outsoles are made from a variety of materials. Properties of the outsole include grip, durability, and water resistance.

Pitch – This is the curve under the heel.

Puff – Reinforcement inside the upper that gives the toe its shape and support; similar in function to a toe cap.

Quarter – This is the back of the shoe where it touches your foot. If it is too low, it will not offer support; if it is too high, it will dig into your ankle.

Seat – This is the top of the heel that touches the upper and sits in the shoe; this is typically shaped to match the form of the upper.

Shank – The curve of the shoe under the arch. The shank absorbs your body weight through the ball of your foot and across the top of your foot. Quality of material here is very important for comfort. Also, a piece of metal inserted between the sole and the insole, lying against the arch of the foot.

Sole – The entire part of the shoe that sits below the wearer's foot, as opposed to the upper. The upper and sole make up the whole of the shoe.

Throat – The front of the vamp next to the toe cap. For shoes where the vamp and quarter panels are one piece, the throat is at the eye-stay.

Toe Box – This is where your toes sit and can be pointy, round, or square. The shoe you pick should complement your height and body type. No matter how pointy the toe box is, you need to be able to wiggle your toes.

Toe Cap – Shoes may have a toe cap in the front upper of the shoe. Toe caps can take various forms, but the distinct types are:

- Complete replacements for the front upper of the shoe
- Stitched-over toe caps that add an extra layer to the upper
- Solid toe caps for protection, such as steel toe caps
- Stitched-over toe caps may be decorative in nature. Toe caps help add strength to the upper front of the shoe, an area that receives a lot of stress and wear from use.

Top Piece – The part of the heel that comes in contact with the ground. It is commonly made of a durable material that helps maintain friction with the ground.

Topline – The top edge of the upper.

Upper – The entire part of the shoe that covers the foot.

Vamp – This is how high or low a shoe is cut along the toes. The higher the vamp, the more support there is, which also helps to keep your foot in position so that it does not slide back and forth. Especially with high heels, it is important to have a high vamp.

Waist – The arch and instep of the foot.

Welt – A strip of material that joins the upper to the sole.

Chapter Note:

1.   http://www.brainyquote.com/quotes/quotes/m/manoloblah387707.html

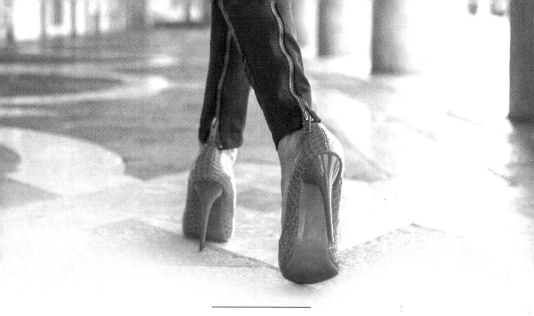

CHAPTER 5

Shopping for Your Sole Mate

"Cinderella ... proof that a new pair
of shoes can change your life."

Many women are crazy about shoes. We love our shoes! Finding the right shoe makes any girl smile and feel giddy inside. I think there is such a special connection between women and their shoes, especially when we find the right shoe that fits, looks good, and is the right price.

Whether you like flat shoes or high-heeled shoes, it is safe to say that a shoe store is like a woman's toy store. It is also safe to say

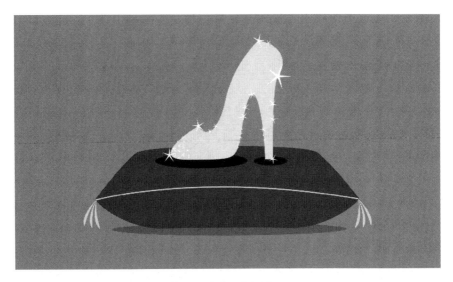

Fig. 17. *Cinderella's Shoes*

that wearing the right shoe makes a *whole* outfit. My dress size has changed so much throughout my life, but my shoe size has stayed the same no matter what dress size I am in at the moment.

It is very important to emphasize that the shoe has to fit your feet: your feet should not adjust to the shoes. No matter how cute the shoes are, if they are not the right fit, let them go—no matter what bargain price they are listed at. I daresay that most women would choose shoes purely for aesthetics and bargain price without considering both comfort and proper fit. This book seeks to instruct buyers to achieve all of these goals by learning the sexy art of high heel shopping. Wearing comfortable and beautiful shoes that fit perfectly can prevent many foot ailments and undue suffering and pain, and may improve balance and wellness as well. This is what I hope for my readers.

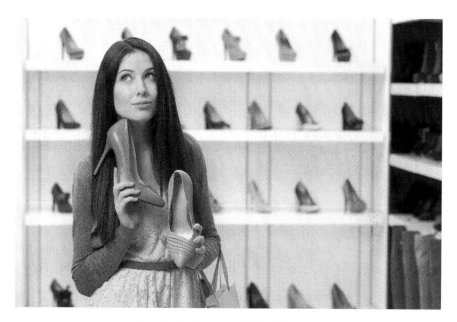

Fig. 18. *The Sexy Art of Shoe Shopping*

THE SEXY ART OF SHOE SHOPPING:

1. There's a right time for shoe shopping.

The best time to measure your foot size is at the *end of the day* because it is the time when feet are at their largest after having expanded or swelled during the day. Measuring feet at the end of the day before buying shoes is ideal because shoe size changes throughout the course of the day.

2. Wear the right size, because size matters.

The majority of people have one foot that is slightly larger than the other, so always try on new shoes on both feet—the shoe has to accommodate the larger foot. Feet have a tendency to swell after wearing shoes for an extended period. If heels are extra snug to begin with, then the wearer will surely be in trouble after a few hours of wear. The last things you want are ingrown toenails or bunions due to a shoe fit that is too tight.

3. Always try the shoe on.

The size marked inside the shoe is not necessarily correct. Shoe sizes are not universally agreed upon. They vary depending on the shoe manufacturer, basic shoe material, and style. A shoe may not necessarily fit the same way depending on the style, brand, and the make of the shoe. The European shoe size system is based on the two-digit system, and the same scale is used for both men and women. The rest of the world, in contrast, has a separate shoe sizing system for males and females. It is very important that you wear the proper shoe size.

There is an international shoe size conversion table for men, women, girls, and boys. Conversion tables are available for American, Australian, British, Canadian, European, Japanese, Korean, Mexican, Russian, Ukrainian, and New Zealanders, in inches, centimeters, and midpoint shoe sizes. These shoe size conversion tables can help. One can use them to convert from the shoe size used in one country or region to the shoe size utilized in another country or region. If you need more information about the international shoe size conversion, you can go to http://www.i18nguy.com/l10n/shoes.html. Store and manufacturer practices regarding returns and exchanges vary widely. This is useful information if you like to shop online.

In a surprising study conducted by the American Orthopedic Foot and Ankle Society and reported on by the Society of Chiropractors and Podiatrists, 88% of women are wearing shoes that are too small for them. That is a pretty staggering figure, and points to a super simple change that can make a huge difference with how one walks in heels. Obviously, wearing properly sized shoes will improve your overall foot health.

4. Knowing your foot shape is very important.

Choose a shoe that is shaped like your foot! During the fitting process, when you are standing up, it is important to allow enough space, approximately ⅜ to ½ inch past your longest toe at the end of each shoe. Ensure that the ball of your foot fits comfortably into the widest part of the shoe.

Do not purchase shoes that feel too tight and expect them to stretch to fit well. If you find that your shoes are a mite too tight, here's a workable solution I use myself: Use a shoe stretcher overnight to shape the shoes to a comfortable width before wearing them.

5. A minimal amount of shoe slipping is allowable.

Your heel should fit comfortably in the shoe; the shoe should not ride up and down on the heel when you walk, causing constant rubbing between your heel skin and the shoe. This friction may cause blisters, swelling, and irritations on the heel area. A bare minimum amount of shoe slipping on the heels is permissible to avoid these painful problems.

6. Try shoes on while standing on a firm surface.

When trying on shoes, be sure to walk on a firm surface like concrete or wooden floor, not carpet, to make sure they fit and feel right and comfortable. Most shoe stores have soft surface flooring on purpose, so that the shoes feel comfortable while you are in the store. When you take home a new pair of shoes, spend some time walking in them to verify that the fit is a good one.

7. The right material matters.

The material for the upper part of the shoe should be made of a soft, flexible material to accommodate the shape and the changes of your foot. Leather is preferable because it reduces the possibility of skin irritations. It will also contour to the shape of your feet over time, which makes the shoe more comfortable to wear, with a fitting like a glove.

8. Sturdy shoes make a difference.

Leather, again, is the preferred material because it is a more durable material than most synthetics. In addition, leather grounds the foot to the floor surface yielding an incredible health benefit (www.earthing.com). Soles that are thick and sustainable provide a solid footing and are not slippery. Thick soles cushion your feet when walking on hard surfaces. Low-heeled shoes are more comfortable, safer, and less demanding than high-heeled shoes. Paper thin shoes do not provide great support for your feet. A rubbery kind of material will absorb foot pressure. If possible, choose a style that is made of a more substantial material.

"You want a thicker sole and a little bit of a platform, which will offset some of the pressure when you are walking."

—DR. CATHERINE MOYER, AS TOLD TO STYLE CASTER

9. Choose a bit of platform.

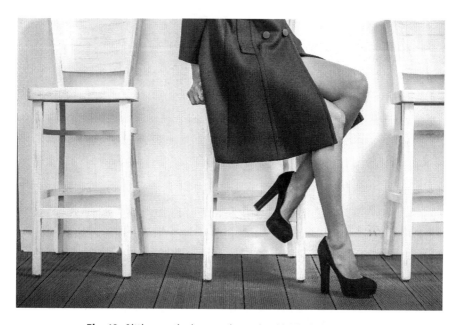

Fig. 19. *Sitting on the bar stool wearing black platform shoes*

The platform reduces the incline of your foot, making things more comfortable all around. The high-heeled shoe that is a strappy, skinny summer stiletto may look like a dream, but it is important to be realistic about what kind of shoe has day-long potential. A thin sole will most likely cause pain for the bottom of your foot. Look for something with some rubber on the bottom to provide a bit of a buffer. What is ideal? A strappy high-heeled shoe with a bit of a platform in the front.

10. Add more cushion.

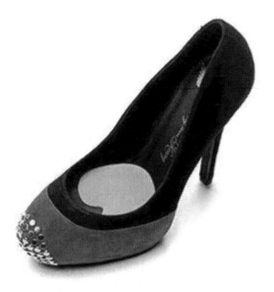

Fig. 20. *Black high heels with pink shoe petals*

Store-bought cushion inserts can be your BFF. Placing additional heel cushion inserts under the balls of your feet will neutralize the majority of the body-weight impact during high-heeled shoe walking. Add the little extra cushion to your shoes, and your dogs will not be barking as quickly. My go-to heel inserts are the foot petals. I always use Dr. Scholl's shoe inserts to add a little shock absorption and added foot comfort in all my high-heeled shoes. Ninety percent of my high-heeled shoes need inserts in order for me to be able to wear them all day at work.

11. Go for a chunky heel: a stacked heel or wedge.

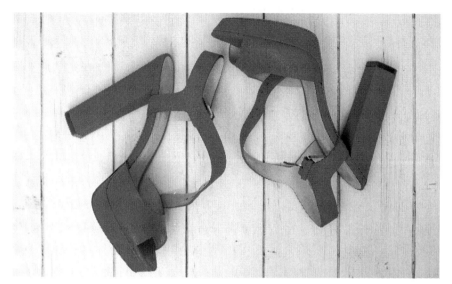

Fig. 21. *Red strappy platform sandals with stacked heels*

The narrower the heel, the greater the pain. So buy a chunkier heel like the stacked heel or a wedge. My favorite work high heels are the three inches stacked heels with ankle straps. I think they are more comfortable and have a sexier look than other high heel options. Podiatrist Erica Schwartz tells *The Washington Post*, "The bigger the heel if it is chunky or a wedge seems to be better because the shoe has a wider base of stability. A skinnier heel and you are more likely to have ankle sprain."

12. Break in the bottoms.

Jay Alexander gave another tip to Glamour Magazine, "Scratch the bottom of your soles with sandpaper." It seems like a strange idea to purposely rough up a brand new pair of shoes, but slick shoes do not provide any traction on smooth surfaces such as hardwood and tile. To resolve the poor traction problem, scuff the soles up a bit. If you do not have sandpaper, stroll up and down a cement sidewalk instead of manually scoring the shoe.

13. Break in your shoes.

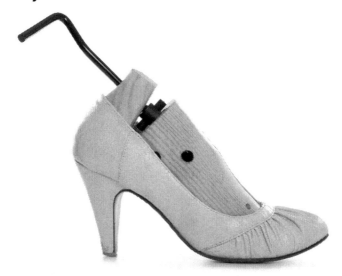

Fig. 22. *Wooden shoe stretcher*

You can use a shoe stretcher or, if possible, manually bend the front of your shoes at least thirty times before wearing them. Breaking in a new pair with a shoe stretcher will increase the width of the shoes. Bending the shoes by hand is like breaking in the shoes without taxing your feet. It is preparing the footwear to be able to accommodate a comfortable feel when you wear the shoes for the first time. Manual bending will enhance the flexibility of the shoes, thus preventing blisters on the sides of your feet, and also allowing for foot expansion at the end of the day, or as you wear your high-heeled shoes for a few hours. Manual bending may not be possible for wedge or platform shoes which tend to be of stiffer construction.

14. Check the heel placement.

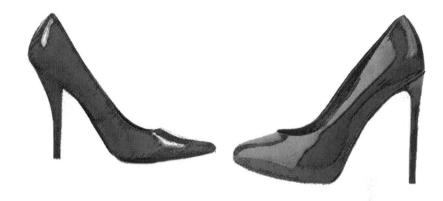

Fig. 23. *Red high heels shoes heel placement*

This is especially critical when choosing thin skinny high heels like stilettos. Choose shoes with heels placed directly under the center of your foot's heel (see photo at left), not at the very back of the shoe (right). This high heel placement is the most efficient way of attaining strong heel support. The heel should be located in the center of the biggest bone (the Calcaneus bone) on your foot. The calcaneus bone carries approximately 100% of the body weight when the heel strikes the ground while walking. The high-heel shock-absorbing load is distributed directly to the ground, instead of to your feet.

15. Get strappy.

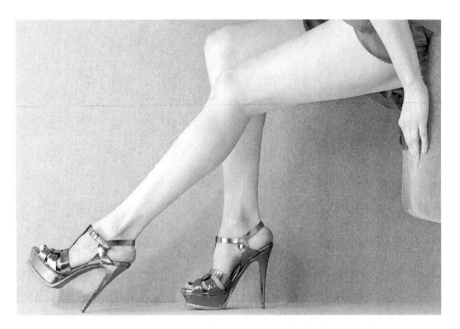

Fig. 24. *Gold strappy platform high heels*

Heels are more comfortable to walk in when you get extra support from straps, such as those found in ballet slippers, Mary Janes, gladiators, or a T-strap shoe. The strap will help to keep the high heels in a secured position because the foot muscles don't have to work as hard to stay in the shoe while walking. Wearing strappy shoes is a particularly good idea when attending a long event, or when lots of walking and dancing are involved.

16. Pace yourself.

If you decide to try high heels for the first time, start with a two-inch wedge. Use baby steps with correct skill set until you build your confidence and master the sexy art of high heel walking technique. If you have never walked in high heels before, do not start out learning in five-inch stilettos—that is a recipe for pain and possibly even injury. College fashion editor Zephyr Basine writes, "Try something smaller like a two-inch heel or wedge to get used to the feeling until your balance has improved. You can always work your way up to your most killer heels once you master the sexy art of high heel walking."[1]

Chapter Note

1.   https://www.bustle.com/articles/33359-how-to-walk-better-in-heels-in-9-easy-tips

MASTERING THE SEXY ART OF HIGH HEEL WALKING

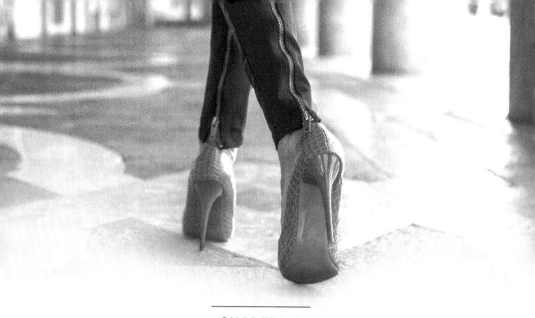

CHAPTER 6

Posture, Posture, Posture!

"A good stance and posture reflect a proper state of mind."

-MORIHEI UESHIBA

Posture is an internal experience. Proper standing posture needs to be felt. Internal posture requires constant self-awareness—the key for a good posture whether you are standing or sitting. It is an internal sensory thing. One needs to be able to recreate posture by feeling it internally with your eyes closed. Visual input has to be minimized, because you will have a tendency to overcorrect yourself. Mirrors are not necessary to keep your posture upright. Your body has an innate divine intelligence of what a properly aligned posture feels like.

NO EFFORT ZONE

When the body is in perfect alignment with gravity, it is in the **No Effort Zone**. No effort for your spine, no effort for your muscles, and no effort for your internal organs, which combined effect allows for the perfect shock absorption capability—especially no effort for your blood circulation. Your heart will be able to pump blood out and bring it back in to replenish without effort.

It is also crucial to note that any minor deviation from this perfect alignment will increase the burden to the body's skeletal system tenfold, while the burden increases to your internal organs exponentially... maybe even a hundred fold!

POSTURE IMPACTS OVERALL BLOOD CIRCULATION

Imagine a garden hose with a kink; it is hard for the water to flow and the water supply will be markedly reduced. Eventually, it will weaken the walls of the garden hose. The same is true with veins and arteries. If there is a kink in the flow, it will impede the circulation of oxygen and nutrients to the rest of the body. Consequently, the body's functions will become inefficient and will have difficulty replenishing internal organs and cells.

HEAD BALANCING ON A STICK, LIKE A GOLF BALL ON A TEE

It is interesting to note that the human head is held only by delicate neck bones and neck muscles in proper balance. Your overall head weight is almost one-fifth of your body weight when you

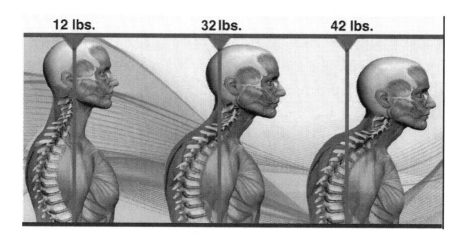

Fig. 25. *Downward Pressure Loading on Three Different Angles of Head Forward Posture[1]*

combine the skull and the brain, not to mention your hair length and hair volume.

Imagine the golf ball on the tee—it is very unstable. If the golf ball is placed improperly on the tee, it will not stay and will fall off. It is mind-boggling to think of how your neck can do all that it does, like tilting your head side to side almost 180 degrees, with the minimal support that it has. Your head is designed to be placed in the middle of the neck ... the head center-balanced position is the most efficient placement of your head.

THE NECK "C" CURVE

There is a reason why there is a reverse "C" curve in the back of your neck, technically called cervical lordosis of the spine. It is a most efficient design to be able to absorb the shock from all of your head weight. It acts as a shock absorber as in a spring mechanism with the disks acting as hydraulics. It is almost the same principle as a suspension bridge. This functional neck reverse "C" curve compensates for the delicate neck muscles and bones.

The neck is loaded with pain sensors in many strategic locations for protection and self-preservation. I think this is so because it can get immediate loving attention from the brain in case there is a weakness in the cervical alignment or a dehydration problem.

The majority of patients I see in my clinic have neck pain. Most of the patients have lost their reverse "C" curve in the neck due to severe muscle spasms and muscle tightness from poor posture and dehydration, combined with poor sleep and stress. The reverse "C" curve and neck muscles are also weakened with constant pillow use at night.

GO PILLOW-LESS

I strongly suggest not using a big, high pillow or, better yet, **no pillow at all** when sleeping at night, because it will strengthen your neck muscles while sleeping. With the support of a pillow, your neck muscles are not activated and not in use. Over time, they will become weak due to disuse. Just think, half of the world does not have a fancy down pillow or a foam pillow, and their necks are stronger, compared to people in the U.S., who have very expensive pillows and yet the greatest incidence of neck pain.

Besides, when lying down while sleeping, the head is supposed to be aligned with the heart on the same level, for ease of blood flow exchange and to allow detox at night during sleep. This position will also enhance cell repair and rejuvenate the rest of the body's internal organs, bones, and muscles.

The blood flow exchange between the heart and the brain is easier when the head is not elevated. Your heart does not have to pump harder against gravity at night when your heart is on the same level as your brain. Most people are used to having pillows for comfort and preference purposes, but it is not correct for optimal brain function and heart circulation.

I suggest slowly teaching yourself to sleep without any pillows until you get used to it. It is good for the neck muscles, for detox, for cell repair, and for recharging purposes. I have many patients who happily told me that after they got used to sleeping without a pillow, their necks became stronger, pain-free, and they slept better too.

HEAD ON A STRING – LIKE A "PUPPET"

To achieve proper head alignment, pretend that your head is held by a vertical string and pulled upward toward the sky by an imaginary active suspension chain. Your ears have to be in alignment with your shoulders. Most people have their head sticking out in front of their shoulders, technically called Upper-crossed Syndrome. This position places an exponential stress load to your whole spine in order to compensate for this forward load.

It is said that every one degree of forwarding tilt increases one pound of load on your neck, and eventually your whole spine. Now, if you add the poor trunk and weak low back posture, the load will increase one hundred times more.

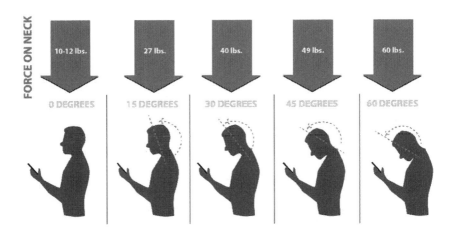

Fig. 26. *Estimation on the Downward Load on the Neck per One Degree of Head Forward Tilt Posture*

The forward head causes most people who are not aware of their head position to feel exhausted at the end of the day. Unbeknownst to them, their body has been working hard fighting gravity with maximum effort due to the poor body alignment and, thus, poor brain circulation. When you add stress, poor diet, and dehydration, the combination becomes the perfect storm for a very exhausting day.

THE RIB CASE

Your trunk is housed and protected by your rib case. (I think it is more accurate to call it a rib case instead of a rib cage ... it is a casing of the vital internal organs, not a prison.) There are an incredible number of pain sensors all over this area which protect the vital organs of your body. The abundance of pain sensors in your rib case is the reason why rib or thoracic injuries are excruciating, because the case is protecting the lungs and heart. Always raise your breast bone to keep your rib case open and to allow your lungs and your heart more room to expand. I always cue the ladies in my clinic to "keep their headlights forward"—that is, both breasts and nipples pointed forward, to maintain the rib case upright.

In your upper back area, it is normal to have a mild hump posture around the rib case. This is technically called Functional Kyphosis in the thoracic area. In plain English, the ribs are shaped like a little barrel, because they enclose the major vital organs, the heart and the lungs. The twelve pairs of ribs attached to the thoracic spine maintain the barrel shape. The stability of the rib bones allows the thoracic area to expand a little and absorb the middle trunk weight efficiently. Any spinal deviation to either side of this point, such as scoliosis, will put constant stress on the vital organs at this level, such as the lungs. If left uncorrected it can eventually cause breathing or respiratory problems, or ultimately heart circulation could be affected, in addition to possibly causing constant mid-thoracic and lower back pain.

THE TWIN SCAPULAR BLADES

There are two scapular blades located on each side of the back rib cage—your shoulder blades. They are held down by several thin, durable layers of mid-scapular muscles and tendons. When there is muscle weakness in the middle muscles between the two shoulder blades, it can cause winging of the scapula, where your rotator cuff muscles and your neck muscles are connected. The winging of the scapula can put a stress load on your neck (cervical spine) because it forces both shoulders to roll forward, and the middle (spinal) border of the scapula lies away from the midline, like an "open book position." Physiologically, the scapula is supposed to be pinned down in the middle upper back, hanging freely. This position allows for efficient rotational gliding, which leaves both shoulder joints free for 360-degree movements.

Poor sitting posture can cause a lot of neck pain, as I have seen in most of my patients. Poor computer-sitting posture is the number one cause of constant neck pain. Ideally, both shoulders should be hanging effortlessly on the side of the back rib case. They should be aligned with your ears when sitting, standing, and lying down.

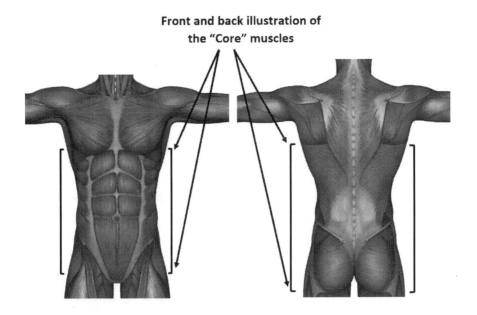

Front and back illustration of the "Core" muscles

Fig. 27. *Front and Back Core Muscles*

THE INTERNAL CORSET-YOUR BACK MUSCLES AND FRONT MUSCLES

Think about it logically, the biggest muscle groups in the body are the core and gluteus muscles (your bum muscles). The lumbar spine (your lower back area) has the reverse C-curve like the C-curve in the neck muscles. This reverse C-curve in your lower back is called lumbar lordosis. It is the most efficient shock-absorbing angle for the spine. It is designed for weight bearing in standing and in walking or in any upright posture.

The abdominal core muscles together with the rib case hold the internal digestive organs in the abdominal cavity. That is why even when you walk, run, or move, these important organs are always in place, held together with the tendons and ligaments in the abdominal area.

Your back core muscles and spinal column are mainly responsible for working with gravity to keep you upright. When you are activating your core muscles, you are wearing the strongest lumbosacral/back corset that God designed you to have. It is inside you, and all you have to do is to activate it. Imagine that every time you tuck your belly button towards your spine, you have tightened the laces of your spinal corset, and you have made it one hundred times stronger.

This corset will intelligently adjust to whatever your activity is and efficiently compensate for you. All you have to do is help by constantly keeping proper posture in sitting, standing, walking, or even running. When your spine is in optimal alignment, you will notice that your feet feel light and most of your body weight is held in the abdominal core area by activating your core and gluteal muscles.

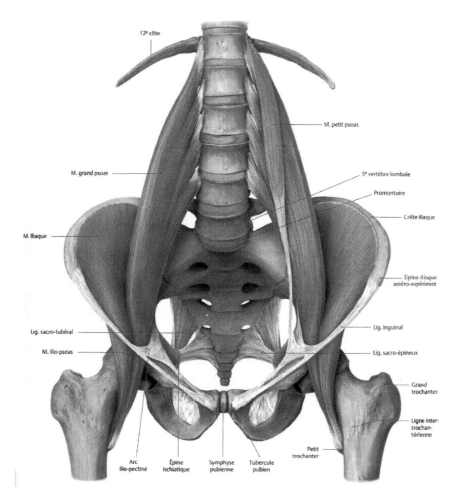

Fig. 28. *Deep Core Muscles–Iliopsoas Muscles*

THE SUPPORT CABLES

Your core muscles function just like the supporting cables of a suspension bridge—an example I use for my patients, so they will be able to appreciate and cue themselves internally. Your spine is the bridge. To keep your spine upright and working efficiently, it has to resist gravity and lateral wind shear regularly.

It has to be vertical for spinal support while it is anchored to the ground. Those vertical structural supports are our core muscles like the iliopsoas muscles, quadratus lumborum, spinal extensors, spinal flexor muscles, and other extensive muscles surrounding the spine, along with several hundreds of tendons and ligaments. Each cell has an innate muscle cell memory for its optimal location.

If, by chance, any of the supporting structures are weakened or are not in the proper alignment, the suspension bridge will lean toward the weakest support and eventually the suspension bridge will collapse to the ground. But before it falls to the ground, it causes so much tension that it increases the workload for the whole system that is trying to keep upright.

Gravity is a fact—a living force on Earth, and human beings were created to be able to work with gravity. Our spinal column is innately designed with proper alignment to absorb the gravitational downward pull of our body weight efficiently. It has amazing, stackable sturdy spinal vertebrae with shock absorbing disc sandwiched in between them. These amazing spinal bones protect your spinal cord by surrounding it with structurally continuous protective rings of solid bone, as well as a complex web of muscles, ligaments, and tendons behind the massive vertebral bone. This rubber-like discs give your spine the flexibility and the shock absorbing capabilities.

This fantastic spinal column design gives each human being the ability to adapt to any posture and the transitional skills needed to survive. In the computer age, the human body has to perform functions that make it challenging to keep upright. The spine is primarily designed for locomotion or walking. It is most tested in sitting positions.

When upright or walking, all of one's body weight is primarily absorbed in the spine, and the majority of the load is carried in the pelvis bone. Think about it; this is the reason why women can carry babies in their abdomens—the amazing pubic bones and muscles have weight-bearing capacity. It has a solid ring design to evenly absorb almost ⅔ of one's body weight and hold all the internal organs in place, while allowing locomotion and adapting to all our movements.

YOUR AMAZING KNEES

Now we will discuss the knees. Together, your thigh bones and pelvic muscles share the weight-bearing duties of your lower half. It is critical that you activate your hip muscles when standing, because the gluteal muscles are attached to them. This weight-bearing system can carry your static weight or stationary weight efficiently this way.

When the gluteal muscles are activated, the leg muscles can move freely and keep one's posture upright above the ground. The knees can function efficiently when the back and thigh muscles are at maximum length, in an isometric and tightened state.

Knees have excellent shock-absorbing cushions like the meniscus and the strong fibrous cartilage sandwiched between the two strong upper and lower leg bones. The knees are also supported by a network of tendons and ligaments that are a powerful suspension system, with all the parts converging in a grand central station network of strong ligaments and tendons around the knee caps. The knee cap is the floating suspension support for the knee. It allows smooth, coordinated knee motion without compromising stability. Most muscles in the knees are coming from both from the hip joint and from the lower leg area such as the strong calf muscles. The knee has an overlapping tendon design which reinforces stability and strength at the same time. The knee is intended to absorb stationary or moving body weight. Your knees have the capacity to absorb three times your body weight when walking, and five times your body weight when running. It is important to note that every pound over the ideal body weight adds five to seven times the stress onto the cartilage and leg bones at the knee junction. The stressed lower leg bones are evident in overweight and obese individuals—their knees are the first thing that wears down, also medically known as osteoarthritis of the knee.

Place all of your weight on the biggest lower leg bones, the tibiae. They connect to your ankles in the back of the feet. You should be able to raise your toes without losing your balance when you put your weight on the back of your heel. This is how you would know that you are putting your weight on the heels and not on your toes – if you can do it without losing your balance.

YOUR FEET AND TOES

Discussing foot anatomy and function is important. You will realize the foot is an amazing design and complex structure if you consider how much it does for the human body. It has a basic composition of

26 small but strong bones, 33 joints, and an efficient and dynamic layer of 120 muscles, ligaments, and nerves.

The foot has several functions in supporting body weight, whether the body is at rest or in motion; it acts as a shock absorber when walking and standing. It works as a lever to move the leg forward during walking, and it also helps maintain balance by adjusting the body to uneven surfaces. It grounds the human body to the earth. It is amazing that though the foot is small in size compared with the rest of the body, each step exerts tremendous force upon the foot. The foot is very dependent on the proper alignment of the spine and its relationship to the rest of the lower extremities during stationary standing and good walking technique.

Your small toe bones are not for weight bearing but instead are used as sensory antennae and balance. Logically, all the bones of your toes are tiny and fragile. They are not designed to carry all of your body weight. I believe that your foot is intended as a fantastic, efficient antenna to the environment.

Your heel bone, also called the calcaneus bone, is the strongest bone in your foot. It is expected to carry and absorb all your body weight whether standing or walking. The impact that force exerts onto the heel and the rest of the foot on average is more than 50% of the body weight during walking and five to seven times more during running. Your feet are extremely narrow relative to your body. As an engineering design, feet defy the basic structural ratio between height and foundation. I wonder why we do not topple over. A typical day equals an average of 4 hours of standing on your feet and a total of 8,000–10,000 steps. That means that the feet support a combined force of several hundred tons every day. Your feet are designed to carry the force of the load efficiently when barefoot.

Your feet have a very comprehensive and extensive network of nerves and circulation, more than your spine and brain combined. Your big toe carries almost 45% of your body's balance sensors. Your toes are the most efficient proprioception and balance sensors. They tell you where the ends of your body and all your joints are located. In Oriental medicine, the feet are believed to be great sensory satellites to all of your internal organs as well as to your immune system. The feet have an extensive network of pain and several sensory satellites like proprioception nerves for balance.

The bottoms of your feet serve as very efficient antennae that are designed to have direct input from Mother Earth. When the foot hits the ground, there are complex neural and muscular interactions happening at nanosecond speed. For example, there is a biofeedback loop to the brain via the spine to keep a person from falling flat on her face while standing or walking. It is amazing how the feet can pull off the bipedal locomotion that walking is, let alone successfully walk on high-heeled shoes.

PROPRIOCEPTION / BALANCE

Proprioception (prō-prē-ō-ˈsep-shən)[2] sounds like a complicated medical term and very technical word. But don't worry, after you read this section, you will have a greater appreciation of proprioception. It has a critical role in balance in both stationary (static) or moving (dynamic) standing balance. I'm sure you are familiar with all the other five senses: touch, taste, hearing, vision, and smell. The sixth sense is the proprioception sense.

In humans, the proprioceptors (muscle spindles) are located in skeletal muscles and tendons (the Golgi tendon organ) and in the fibrous capsules in your joints. They are responsible for telling the brain the location of all joints and extremities without looking. They are different from the exteroceptors that help you sense the outside world, or the interoceptors that help you feel pain, hunger, and the movement of internal organs, et cetera.

The brain translates all information from proprioceptors and the vestibular system located in your inner ear into its overall sense of body position, motion, and acceleration. The word kinesthesia (kinesthetic sense) strictly means movement sense, but has been used inconsistently to refer either to proprioception alone or to the brain's interpretation of the messages from the proprioceptors and vestibular inputs. All of the other primary senses have to develop before proprioception sense is gained. Proprioception sense is the last to fully develop, as a child becomes mobile—senses like sight, hearing, and smell come quickly after birth. It is the proprioceptors that tell the body about a joint position location. Proprioception has unconscious (right reflex) and conscious (postural and balance) parts. It is the unconscious sense of movement of your arms and legs and where they are, without looking or without the need of visual input.

It is important to emphasize the significance of the soles of your feet. They contain an extensive sensory system designed with a massive network of nerves and sensory receptors—more than the spinal cord and brain combined. When barefoot, the soles are the body's primary connection to Mother Earth, providing biofeedback for proprioception and balance.

When a baby starts to grow and develop proprioceptors, it first develops in the neck for head control. The baby will start holding its head upright. Then, the baby will start rolling from side to side, sitting, and finally crawling. It will have fully developed proprioceptors in all the joints and muscles. These steps contribute to achieving a good static balance and dynamic standing balance, which will then lead to beginner walking skills such as cruising across furniture and the ability to stand in an upright posture. Eventually, as the child grows to maturity, the skills of walking and running are mastered.

It is a fact that the proprioception sense is damaged whenever the body incurs an injury to the legs, particularly injuries to the foot or ankle. It could be interrupted by injuries such as a fracture, sprain, strain, overuse, swelling, inflammation, or just by more than two days of bed rest, or by any chronic degenerative disease progression. Proprioception is also slow to be restored or rehabilitated after injury. Poorly healed ankle or foot proprioceptors are the number one cause of foot and ankle re-injuries, when the sense of proprioception is not restored during recovery.

As we get older, we do not pay attention to maintaining and improving both our static (stationary) and dynamic (moving) standing balance. Over time one's standing balance deteriorates, if left unattended. Poor balance is the number one cause of most geriatric fall accidents. Just like any other body part, proprioception sense and balance have to be regularly maintained and improved by incorporating them into your daily exercise program. The proprioceptive sense can be sharpened through study of multiple balance disciplines such as balance boards, Pilates, exercise balls, dancing, or any movement activity of your choice.

The fastest way to improve your proprioception and balance is by challenging it. First, perform your usual exercise program by adding a blindfold to the routine and, preferably, go barefoot! Your brain will be forced to utilize your internal proprioceptors efficiently in your joints, particularly in your feet and ankles.

Another radical way of challenging your proprioception is by wearing high-heeled shoes. Learning proper high heel standing posture and correct high heel walking technique is guaranteed to significantly improve your proprioceptors. Wearing high heels

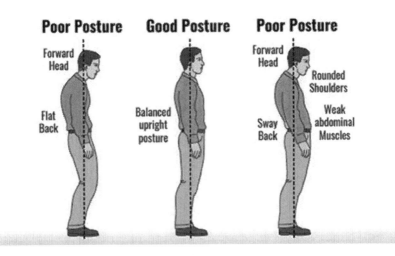

Fig. 29. *Illustration of the Comparison between Good Posture and Bad Posture*

will also enhance and continually challenge your stationary and moving standing balance. High heel walking is a fun and efficient way to maintain your overall stationary and moving standing balance.

THE TWELVE EASY POINTS FOR PROPER UPRIGHT STANDING POSTURE

To achieve the sexy art of high heel walking, it is important first to master the proper upright standing posture barefoot. One has to know how to internally feel a proper postural body alignment. Mastering barefoot standing is the basic foundational knowledge of the sexy art of high heel walking. To make it easy for the reader, I have created graphic illustrations and a quick list of twelve easy steps for learning correct posture. First practice the proper standing upright posture barefoot until you have mastered it.

1. Barefoot, stand with your legs hip-width apart, eyes closed. If you happen to feel dizzy or have vertigo when your eyes are closed, make sure you stand next to a wall for safety, to keep you from falling if you lose your balance.
2. Imagine the vertebrae of your spine as stacked one on top of the other from your lower back up to the neck bones.
3. Imagine you are a puppet, and a string is attached to the top of your head, pulling upward to the sky. Elongate all levels of your spine upward. Feel the sensation that your neck is being pulled upward. Feel the spaces between your neck bones expanding. Relax your neck and jaw.

4. Make sure your ears are in alignment with your shoulders, and your chin is tucked back, while your head is at a neutral angle.

5. Keep the breastbone raised up. Pretend like you are pulling up a necktie, with both breasts and nipples pointing forward like headlights on a car. (I used to joke with my patients: Ladies, aim your headlights forward!)

6. Both shoulder blades in your back are almost squeezed together, pointed and slid downward ... relaxed.

7. Take a deep breath quietly while expanding your upper rib cage (inhale and exhale with mouth closed). Keep the jaw relaxed and the tongue gently touching the front roof of the mouth.

8. Tuck or pull your belly button toward your spine. Engaging the core muscles is a better way of activating your deep spinal muscles. Imagine that you are tightening your internal lumbar corset.

9. Tuck (engage) your lower core muscles. Imagine you are zipping your pants while still able to breathe and expand your upper rib cage.

10. Tighten your gluteal muscles (your bum muscles), alternating one at a time while standing.

11. Lock or straighten both knees, and tighten the quadriceps, the front muscles of your thighs.

12. Put your weight on your heels, using the biggest bone in your leg and ankle to carry your body weight, and unload your front feet. Your toes are relaxed while still flat on the floor, with minimal weight on your toes.

Please master this basic and most essential foundation of your proper standing posture barefoot before going on to the next chapter ... the sexy art of high heel walking!

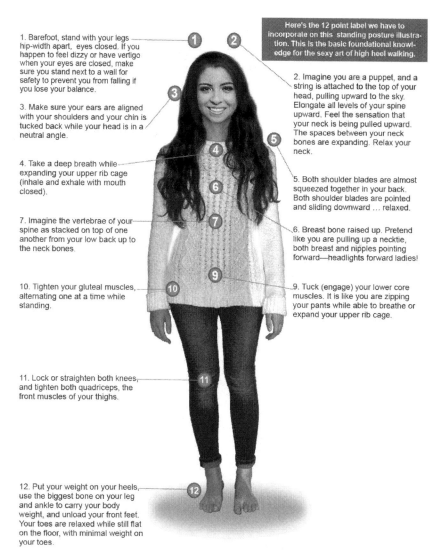

Here's the 12 point label we have to incorporate on this standing posture illustration. This is the basic foundational knowledge for the sexy art of high heel walking.

1. Barefoot, stand with your legs hip-width apart, eyes closed. If you happen to feel dizzy or have vertigo when your eyes are closed, make sure you stand next to a wall for safety to prevent you from falling if you lose your balance.

2. Imagine you are a puppet, and a string is attached to the top of your head, pulling upward to the sky. Elongate all levels of your spine upward. Feel the sensation that your neck is being pulled upward. The spaces between your neck bones are expanding. Relax your neck.

3. Make sure your ears are aligned with your shoulders and your chin is tucked back while your head is in a neutral angle.

4. Take a deep breath while expanding your upper rib cage (inhale and exhale with mouth closed).

5. Both shoulder blades are almost squeezed together in your back. Both shoulder blades are pointed and sliding downward ... relaxed.

6. Breast bone raised up. Pretend like you are pulling up a necktie, both breast and nipples pointing forward—headlights forward ladies!

7. Imagine the vertebrae of your spine as stacked on top of one another from your low back up to the neck bones.

9. Tuck (engage) your lower core muscles. It is like you are zipping your pants while able to breathe or expand your upper rib cage.

10. Tighten your gluteal muscles, alternating one at a time while standing.

11. Lock or straighten both knees, and tighten both quadriceps, the front muscles of your thighs.

12. Put your weight on your heels, use the biggest bone on your leg and ankle to carry your body weight, and unload your front feet. Your toes are relaxed while still flat on the floor, with minimal weight on your toes.

Fig. 30. *Standing Posture Barefoot Front*

Chapter Notes

1. www.ericdalton.com
2. Webster dictionary

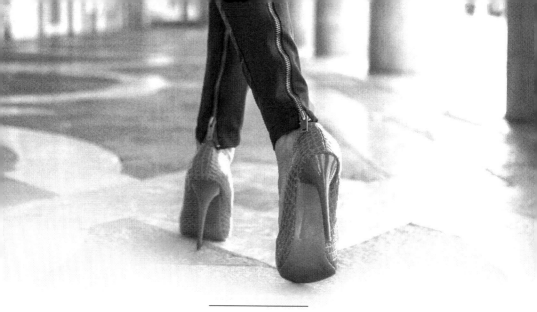

CHAPTER 7

Take a Step with Your High Heels

"A shoe has so much more to
offer than just to walk."

-CHRISTIAN LOUBOUTIN

It is essential to master proper upright standing posture barefoot before putting on high-heeled shoes. Please review and master the posture chapter. Don't forget the shoe cushions before putting on the high heels. Now let's get on to the sexy art of high heel walking ... are you ready?

Here are the step-by-step details for proper standing posture in high-heeled shoes.

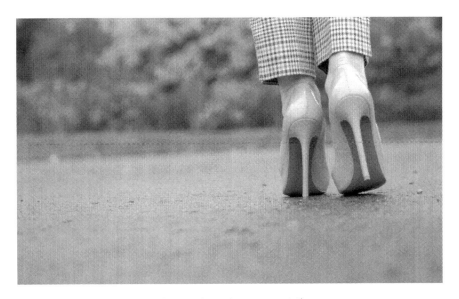

Fig. 31. *The Red Bottom Louis'* [1]

1. Do a mental review of the 12-point checklist of the proper upright posture while barefoot on the ground.

2. Put on your high-heeled shoes. Reset your standing posture while on the shoes. Readjust your upright posture because your body's center of gravity is slightly elevated due to the high-heeled shoes you are wearing.

3. Review from the head to the toes the proper upright posture while in high-heeled shoes. Then, try the same upright standing posture on high heels with your eyes closed.

4. Check your feet, and make sure that you feel your body weight in your heels, not in your toes.

5. Check your head to spine alignment.

6. Always engage your core muscles, gluteal muscles (your bum muscles), and your leg muscles.

7. Once your upright posture is stable, start by shifting your weight one hip at a time, alternating between hips.

8. Try to contract your gluteal muscles (your bum muscles) while shifting your weight.

9. With your knees locked, tighten your quads on the weight bearing leg, while relaxing the unloaded leg.

10. Start to pick up one heel at a time in place, while slightly bending your knee, just to internalize alternating weight shifting while on your high-heeled shoes.

11. Remember to put all your weight on your heels (the back of the foot), not on your toes.

12. Slightly raise your toes when unloading during weight shifting, to make sure that you are not putting pressure on your toes. Also, this enables you to verify if your dynamic standing balance is very stable.

This list explains how I have stood on my high-heeled shoes for 10 to 14 hour work days for almost 20 years now: weight shifting one leg at a time and raising the toes to unload the sciatic nerve while standing on high heels.

There's another standing pose on high heels: Try to cross your legs at the hip level while standing. Your body weight will be evenly distributed across your pelvic bones with a more stable cross-legged stance. Try this position. It is easy on the back and feet and, besides, it looks sexy!

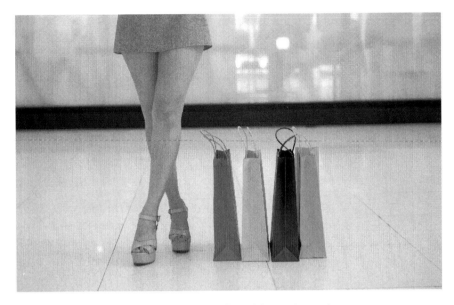

Fig. 33. *Static Standing with Legs Crossed*

THE ULTIMATE POWER WALK

WALKING IN HIGH HEELS PAIN-FREE WITH GRACE AND CONFIDENCE.

"Your foot wears the shoe, instead of the shoe wearing you."

—DR. VALERIE YOUNGBLOOD, MD

Like learning any new skill, mastering the sexy art of high heel walking requires the right shoes for your skill level. A few practical measures like proper standing postures, patience, and practice are critical at this point. Practice until it becomes second nature. Practice until your high-heeled shoes become an extension of your body.

According to neuro-learning theory, before a new skill is considered established and mastered in your brain, it has to be repeated at least five thousand times. PRACTICE! PRACTICE! PRACTICE!

Review your standing posture foundation and your proper upright posture with high-heeled shoes on. Check your balance, engage your core muscles, and activate your internal corset. Now, ready to walk?

Here are the twelve important cues of the sexy art of high heel walking!

1. Always start with the proper standing posture on high heels.

(Assuming that you have reviewed and mastered the proper standing posture on high heels.)

2. Lead with the Core Muscles

When you walk, lead with your core muscles while they are in constant activation.

3. Move Your Entire Leg, Hip, and Thighs Forward All Together

Keep one foot forward, landing on your heel first, while tightening your gluteal muscles.

4. Hip Sway Sideways

Exaggerate your hip's sideways sway to clear the foot off the ground. This will compensate for the restricted ankle joint flexibility caused by the high-heeled shoes.

5. Keep Your Knee Straight by Tightening Quads

As the foot hits the ground, keep the advancing leg and knee straight. Bended knees look goofy with high heels! Again, the exaggerated hip sway is sufficient to compensate for the restricted ankle joint movement, because your foot is in a continually pointed toe, lengthened position. The heel elevation from the high-heeled shoe is the primary driver for the particular walking technique required.

6. Lead with the Knee on the Advancing Leg

This is the other foot that is behind you. Bend your knee while advancing the same leg forward. Your foot will gracefully follow behind the knee.

7. Controlled Heel Landing

Intentionally control your heel landing. Try to land your feet quietly and gently like a cool cat. This is achieved by continuously activating your core muscles and an exaggerated hip sway to the side. Be mindful on each step. When your foot lands intentionally softly, it is gentle to your foot bones and muscles. You will find yourself putting less pressure on the balls of the feet this way.

8. Comfortable Arm Swing

Swing your arm on the alternating side from the foot to project a more relaxed and confident high-heeled walk.

9. Take Smaller Steps

Make sure to take a comfortable stride length, not too big, not too small of a step, just enough distance that you can maintain your posture and balance. Too big or too small of a step will disrupt your posture and balance. Wearing high heels automatically makes your stride shorter, so you will need to take more graceful, smaller steps than usual.

10. Be Confident - Own Your Ultimate Power Walk

With proper high heel walking technique, walking will feel like you are gliding with your shoes across the floor. Walk with grace and confidence. Wearing high heels properly and confidently means you are making your presence known as you glide with your high-heeled shoes. Walk as if you have just been declared the winner of a beauty pageant. Occupy the space you are walking in, and SMILE! It is not sexy when a lady is suffering while wearing her high-heeled shoes.

11. Slow It Down

High-heeled shoes are not worn in gym class for a reason, so take your time when you are walking in them. Zephyr Basine wrote on college fashion, "Don't expect to be able to walk as fast as you normally do in high heels."[2]

12. Take Breaks

Whether you are wearing heels or not, being on your feet for an extended period will hurt your feet. Do yourself a favor and take turns standing and sitting over the course of the day or night.

It is critical to point out that "Runway Walking" is not the same as the sexy art of high heel walking. The technique of runway walking used by supermodels is exaggerated for the purpose of showcasing the fashion clothes they are dramatically presenting. Try not to cross your heels, stepping one foot over the other as is done in runway walking—it is dangerous to do a runway walk on the street.

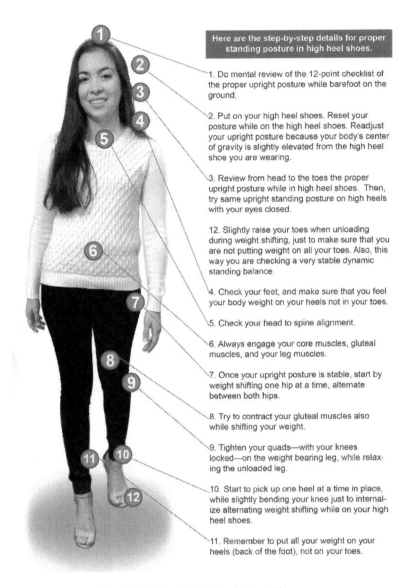

Here are the step-by-step details for proper standing posture in high heel shoes.

1. Do mental review of the 12-point checklist of the proper upright posture while barefoot on the ground.

2. Put on your high heel shoes. Reset your posture while on the high heel shoes. Readjust your upright posture because your body's center of gravity is slightly elevated from the high heel shoe you are wearing.

3. Review from head to the toes the proper upright posture while in high heel shoes. Then, try same upright standing posture on high heels with your eyes closed.

12. Slightly raise your toes when unloading during weight shifting, just to make sure that you are not putting weight on all your toes. Also, this way you are checking a very stable dynamic standing balance.

4. Check your feet, and make sure that you feel your body weight on your heels not in your toes.

5. Check your head to spine alignment.

6. Always engage your core muscles, gluteal muscles, and your leg muscles.

7. Once your upright posture is stable, start by weight shifting one hip at a time, alternate between both hips.

8. Try to contract your gluteal muscles also while shifting your weight.

9. Tighten your quads—with your knees locked—on the weight bearing leg, while relaxing the unloaded leg.

10. Start to pick up one heel at a time in place, while slightly bending your knee just to internalize alternating weight shifting while on your high heel shoes.

11. Remember to put all your weight on your heels (back of the foot), not on your toes.

Fig. 34. *Walking in High Heels Front View*

Chapter Notes

1. http://www.foreveramber.co.uk/2015/05/how-to-walk-in-high-heels-without-pain-and-without-falling-over.html

2. https://www.collegefashion.net/fashion-tips/a-girls-guide-to-high-heels-part-1-how-to-walk-in-heels/Z.Basine

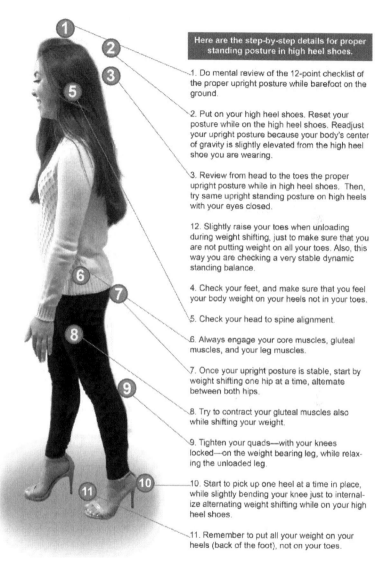

Here are the step-by-step details for proper standing posture in high heel shoes.

1. Do mental review of the 12-point checklist of the proper upright posture while barefoot on the ground.

2. Put on your high heel shoes. Reset your posture while on the high heel shoes. Readjust your upright posture because your body's center of gravity is slightly elevated from the high heel shoe you are wearing.

3. Review from head to the toes the proper upright posture while in high heel shoes. Then, try same upright standing posture on high heels with your eyes closed.

12. Slightly raise your toes when unloading during weight shifting, just to make sure that you are not putting weight on all your toes. Also, this way you are checking a very stable dynamic standing balance.

4. Check your feet, and make sure that you feel your body weight on your heels not in your toes.

5. Check your head to spine alignment.

6. Always engage your core muscles, gluteal muscles, and your leg muscles.

7. Once your upright posture is stable, start by weight shifting one hip at a time, alternate between both hips.

8. Try to contract your gluteal muscles also while shifting your weight.

9. Tighten your quads—with your knees locked—on the weight bearing leg, while relaxing the unloaded leg.

10. Start to pick up one heel at a time in place, while slightly bending your knee just to internalize alternating weight shifting while on your high heel shoes.

11. Remember to put all your weight on your heels (back of the foot), not on your toes.

Fig. 35. *Walking in High Heels Side View*

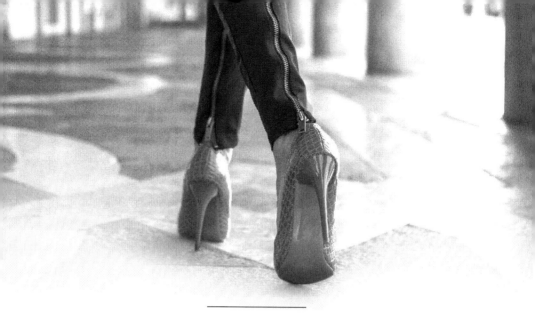

CHAPTER 8

Sitting with Elegance

*"Slouching affects the confidence in your
thought and ability to do your job"*

T he sexy art of high heel walking also involves the sexy art of
proper sitting while wearing high heels. Proper sitting posture
with high heels is essential to master as well, in order to maintain good health and prevent injuries.

The same spinal alignment in good standing posture on heels applies
to the spinal alignment in elegant sitting position in heels, except that
the legs follow the 90/90/90 rule: 90 degrees hip flexion, 90 degrees
of knee flexion, and 90 degrees ankle-neutral position, while resting

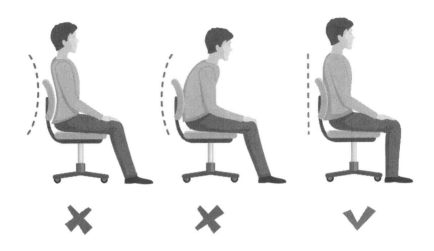

Fig. 36. *Illustrations of Three Sitting Positions On an Office chairs*

comfortably on the floor. However, in sitting in high heels, one has to exaggerate the pelvic bone forward tilt a bit, and point your tailbone backward. This will minimize the urge to dig your tailbone downward in order to keep optimal spine alignment. Don't collapse the spine when sitting. Always be mindful that there is an imaginary string that is pulling your spine upward to maintain upright sitting posture.

The sexy art of proper sitting while on high heels is as follows:

1. When changing from standing to sitting, always put one foot slightly forward of the other.
2. Make sure that the back leg is touching the chair.
3. As you lower yourself into the chair, land gently and gracefully by using the back leg as the primary driver for the whole sitting down motion. Keep the second leg slightly in front of the other.

4. Sit with core muscles always engaged, tucking the belly button to the spine.

5. Maintain an upright posture. Imagine a string pulling your head up at all times. Keep your ears in alignment with your shoulders.

6. Don't lean on the back rest. Place both hands on your lap, palms down, and in relaxed position.

7. To maintain sitting position, keep the knees together at all times. You may cross the ankles or just put the ankles close to each other.

8. To get up from sitting, scoot toward the edge of the chair. Remember to place one foot slightly in front of the other.

9. Slightly lean your head forward, until your nose is just past the knee.

10. Rise up while pushing up with the back leg, all the way to the proper upright posture with heels.

The backrest of a chair is not your friend. It forces your spine to slouch with the chair's backrest, neutralizing all the functional and physiological curvatures of the neck and thoracic and lumbar spine. It is easy to neglect one's posture when sitting in heels, if one leans on the backrest of a chair. It is okay to lean on the backrest for a few seconds at a time, but not for more than five minutes at a time.

Please note that prolonged sitting while leaning on the backrest decreases your blood circulation approximately 50%. It will misalign your posture to lean back continuously while sitting. It is hard to activate your core muscles while slouching on a backrest. Gravity will negatively affect your body because of your poorly activated core muscles.

COMPUTERITIS SYNDROME

In this book, please allow me to mention this modern day silent epidemic ... I think it is important to discuss **COMPUTERITIS SYNDROME**. I invented this word in my Holistic Physical Therapy Clinic. In my practice I see a lot of patients who suffer from this syndrome.

"COMPUTERITIS SYNDROME" is prevalent in young and old alike. It is caused by sustained crooked sitting posture with a

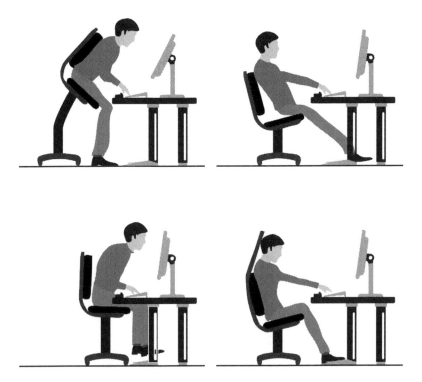

Fig. 37. *Poor Computer Sitting Postures that may cause COMPUTERITIS SYNDROME*

slouched spine resting on the backrest of the chair, while in front of a computer, with one's head and chin protruding forward, and both arms extended forward typing on the keyboard for extended periods of time (particularly for more than thirty minutes).

Assuming this poor sitting position for a prolonged length of time can lead to multiple health problems in a short period of time. **COMPUTERITIS SYNDROME** is a combination of multiple clinical symptoms. Initially, it starts as muscle tightness or spasms in the neck or lower back, mild to moderate neck pain, occipital neuralgia, and mild to moderate lower back pain, headache, TMJ tightness, jaw pain, and fatigue. In more advanced cases, the sufferer has all of the complaints previously mentioned but with intense pain, as well as additional clinical symptoms such as hypertension, depression, metabolic syndrome, insulin resistance, and type 2 diabetes.

Most children and adults use a computer for more than four to eight hours a day. Using a computer, while sitting for more than thirty minutes at a time without standing for few minutes break, is considered hazardous to your health. It is a significant threat to your overall physical and mental health. Health deterioration starts from the head down to your toes.

Starting with the forward head posture, also called Upper Crossed Syndrome, symptoms could include most commonly neck pain, TMJ pain, and headache. In some instances degenerative disk disease develops, also known as disk bulging. This forward head posture will load the front muscle of the neck with 75% of one's head weight, and pull on the back of your neck muscles, leading to severe neck muscle spasms. The eyes will eventually be damaged after prolonged staring at the blue light of the computer screen. The eye muscles can become strained and weakened, resulting in compromised vision such as myopia or other eye problems.

Bad computer posture weakens and collapses your postural muscles, such as the tightening of the iliopsoas muscles, also called Iliopsoas Syndrome. I see this condition frequently in my outpatient physical therapy clinic. Patients present as having one-sided lower back pain, which increases when getting up from a chair or toilet, or when bending, or having difficulty getting in and out of a car. The weakening of the abdominal and spinal core muscles can lead to lower back pain, possible lumbar disk degeneration, and eventually a pinched nerve. Your core muscles are designed to be activated efficiently and continuously by gravity when standing or walking. That is why they are called postural muscles.

Prolonged sitting slows down the functions of the internal organs including the liver, the pancreas, and the heart. They all become sluggish and inefficient. The lungs' ability to fully expand inside the rib case will become restricted over time. The overall blood circulation to body and brain will decrease by approximately 50% to 65%. Some patients will experience constipation due to constriction and compression of the digestive cavity during the prolonged sitting position. Leg circulation will also be affected. Blood and fluids will be pulled into your legs, leading to leg and foot swelling, cramping, and muscle weakness. Your standing balance will also slowly deteriorate, since your feet are not being challenged in the sitting position.

Computer screens emit a constant low level of electromagnetic field (EMF), called "dirty electricity," which will directly impact the electrically charged heart located right in front of the computer monitor. The heart is directly and constantly bombarded with the EMF when one sits in front of the computer monitor. This may affect thyroids and sleep, causing feelings of fatigue and, sometimes, depression.

One's overall physical and mental health are gravely affected over time by prolonged sitting at a computer. The human body was not designed for sitting for more than thirty minutes at a time. I usually tell my patients that God never designed chairs; otherwise, He would have made our tailbones less protruding and pointy, with a smoother pelvic bone design—a better design than what it is.

Another very informative book that I highly recommend is *Sitting Kills, Moving Heals*, written by a NASA head researcher, Dr. Joan Vernikos. In her book, she has proven that sitting for more than thirty minutes at a time is very hazardous to one's health. One needs to stand for at least five minutes for every thirty minutes of sitting position. Human beings are designed to walk and be upright 70% of the time. This is your body's optimal position to function at peak efficiency of all bodily functions including blood circulation.

Prolonged sitting increases your insulin resistance to glucose by 40%, thus leading to type-2 diabetes. Sitting also lowers the function of our fat burning enzymes, increasing chances of weight gain. Extended inactivity, such as prolonged sitting, also promotes muscle breakdown, and gradually decreases your bone mass by 1% per year.

Prolonged sitting also decreases the supply of brain-enhancing hormones, thus causing depression and poor mood. Sitting cuts your heart blood circulation by 54%. It also increases your chances of contracting prostate and breast cancers by 30%. Prolonged sitting, that is, for more than six hours daily, cuts out seven years of good quality life. It is a common practice for Americans to head to the gym after eight hours of sitting, believing that this practice will neutralize the adverse effects of prolonged sitting. Based on recent NASA studies, this is not so. The best way to neutralize the effects is by standing up for five minutes for every thirty minutes of prolonged sitting.

I suggest to patients at my clinic that they use an exercise ball as an office chair.

It activates your core, and there is a counter shock-absorbing upward bounce with the ball. When used as a chair, the exercise ball is gentle on your spine. It also challenges your dynamic sitting balance. There's a company that adopted a chair design for office based on the exercise ball— just search online if you're interested.

Choose the right sized ball for your height to achieve the 90 hip/90 knee/90 ankle position. Bouncing on these exercise balls for at least two minutes or more while sitting will help the spine relax

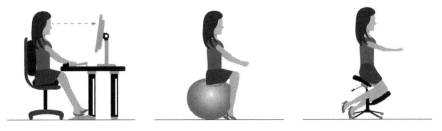

Fig. 38. *Illustrations of Three Good Computer Sitting Postures*

and distribute the force of gravitational pull on the spine, achieving "Zero Effort." Always limit sitting to thirty minutes at a time, even if you are using one of these special office chairs.

How about the expensive "ergonomic chairs"? A chair is a chair ... it doesn't matter if it's ergonomically designed or not, it will still cause COMPUTERITIS SYNDROME. It is important to know that it is not the chair ... it is the prolonged sitting position, more than thirty minutes at a time, day in and day out, that is harmful to your health!

The adjustable standing desk would be ideal also. It gives the individual a flexible work desk that alternates from sitting to standing position in a convenient and efficient way. Changing from sitting to standing every thirty minutes at work will be doable with this standing desk. It would also prevent the development of degenerative diseases and other medical problems resulting from prolonged sitting.

If the standing desk is not an option for you, there is actually a simple solution to this problem. **Get up every for five minutes for every thirty minutes of sitting!** (I am actually doing it while writing this book.) Constantly change your position from sitting to standing and vice versa throughout the day. Prolonged standing is not good for you either!

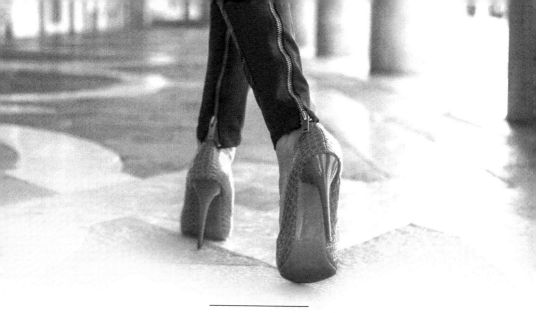

CHAPTER 9

Special Situations

"Sometimes it takes a good fall to know where you really stand."

-HAYLEY WILLIAMS

WALKING ON UNSTABLE SURFACES SUCH AS GRASS, SAND, OR SOFT GROUND

The key to walking in high heels on an unstable ground such as grass or other soft surfaces is to put all of your weight on the ball of your toes, and unload the heels, so that the heels will not sink into the unstable surface. It is a good idea to use high heel expanders or heel protectors for grass walking if you can find some.

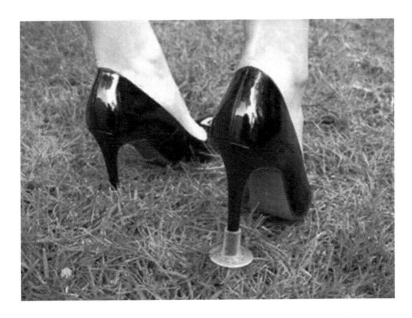

Fig. 39. *High Heel Expanders for Grass or Soft Surface High Heel Walking*[1]

Having good balance will serve you well on these kinds of surfaces. Hanging on to your escort would be ideal to make sure you can maintain the tippy-toe walking. Practically, this is the ONLY situation in which walking on your tiptoes is required. Loading weight on the heels is not a good idea with soft and unstable surfaces.

GETTING IN AND OUT OF A CAR WHEN WEARING HIGH HEELS

To get in a car:

- If possible, first … sit on the car seat sideways.
- With both knees together, pivot toward the inside of the car.
- Bring one leg at a time inside the car and sit facing forward.
- Always keep an upright sitting posture.

- Do not lean too much on the backrest even with a seat belt on.

To get out of the car:

- Keep your knees together.
- Turn both knees out toward the door.
- Safely land both feet on the ground.
- Place one foot slightly in front of the other.
- Push on the one leg slightly behind the other leg to get up gracefully and effortlessly to a proper upright position.

GOING UP STAIRS:

- Always use the hand rail, if one is available.
- Take your time. Don't rush!
- Step up with the front part of the shoe, one at a time.
- Control your landing gracefully, landing the heels quietly, every step of the way.
- Place all of your weight on the balls of your feet, while constantly activating your core muscles.

GOING DOWN STAIRS:

- Always hold onto a rail while wearing high-heeled shoes.
- Place one foot slightly sideways on the stair steps one foot at a time, so you do not feel like gravity is pulling you down.
- Progress slowly and gracefully. Do not rush.
- Always walk on the balls of your feet when walking down stairs.

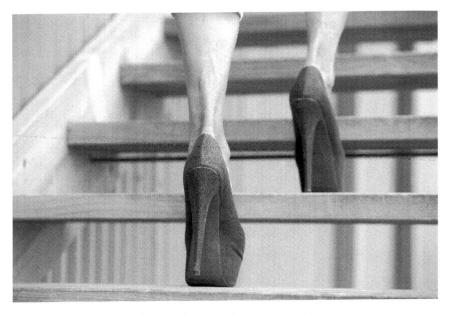

Fig. 40. *High Heels Going Up on Stairs*

IF A FALL HAPPENS

After a fall, do not get up right away! Take your time to recover your bearings and check for injuries. After establishing that there is no damage, take about nine deep breaths to calm yourself, starting with an exhale. This is instinctively what your brain does to cue for stress relief (activating the parasympathetic system). Ask someone to help you up. Most likely your balance will still be off after falling, so it's best not to walk right away. Recover your balance first. Once upright, wait for another nine seconds; again exhale first, to allow your brain to calm down before you take another step. Most people fall a second time immediately after the initial fall. This is because one's sense of equilibrium has not yet recovered from the original trauma of falling.

Rebalance yourself. Take your time. Smile before you take another step. Always recover with grace after a fall.

Chapter Note

1. http://cdn1.bigcommerce.com/server3200/7nf10l43/product_images/theme_images/BlackHAonShoe_01.jpg?t=1477550388

SECTION D

PAMPERING YOUR FEET AND SHOES

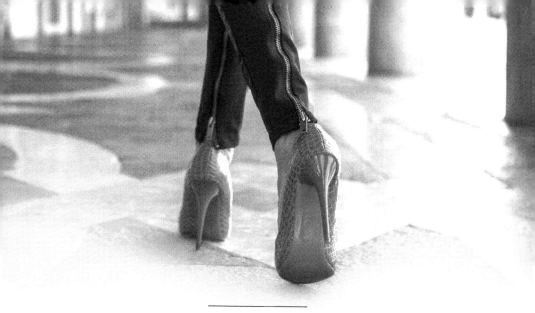

CHAPTER 10

Food for Your Feet

"I can't control everything in my life but I can
control what I put in my body."

The majority of people do not see a connection between the food they eat and their foot health. Yet most painful foot conditions and weaknesses can be prevented or lessened by maintaining a healthy gut with healthy eating habits.

The foot and ankle contain: 26 bones (one-quarter of the bones in the human body are in the feet); 33 joints; more than 100 muscles, tendons, and ligaments; and a network of blood vessels, nerves, skin, and soft tissue. These components work together to provide the entire body with support, balance, and mobility, so we need to keep them active and healthy. This chapter suggests simple but important self-healing concepts that will keep your feet and your entire body healthy and happy.

1. PROPER HYDRATION

Proper hydration is essential. The body is made up of approximately 65-75% saline water. It runs on hydraulics. The heart, lungs, and brain are the primary organs that your body prioritizes and regularly supplies with the much-needed saline water every second of your life. Your leg and foot muscles, bones and joint cartilage, tendons, ligaments, and blood also function through hydraulics. You need to drink half of your body weight in equal ounces daily. Add a pinch of sea salt per eight ounces of filtered water, preferably Himalayan sea salt. Himalayan sea salt contains much needed 80 to 90 micro and macro minerals. I strongly suggest reading the book *Water* by Dr. Batmanghelidj.

Essentially, the body is composed of saline water. Proper hydration is the reason why hospitals always give a patient an IV of saline water when admitted, because it helps the body to heal faster. You don't need to be hospitalized to access this healing saline water. You can make your own at home daily by drinking filtered water with a pinch of Himalayan Sea salt. When the body is fully hydrated, the feet can absorb the body weight better, whether standing or walking throughout the day ... your feet will thank you!

2. ESSENTIAL FATTY ACIDS (EFA)

The tendons, ligaments, and muscles all over the body, particularly in the hips, legs, and feet, all rely primarily on essential fatty acids for strength and shock absorbing qualities. Chapped or cracked heels are a sign that the body lacks EFAs. Applying lotion in such a case is just a superficial Band-Aid—it is not the best way to address the problem. It is best to get the optimal EFAs daily in your diet or through supplements to prevent dry skin and chapped heels.

It is important to note that if your gallbladder has been removed, your body will have difficulty digesting and absorbing EFAs or any kind of fat. In this situation, I suggest you take supplements such as a dietary bile supplement to break down fats and improve the body's absorption of EFAs. Ask a qualified health practitioner in your area about this.

Healthy, good fats in your diet means eating daily the right ratios of omega 3, 6, and 9, plus extra virgin coconut oil, organic lard, organic tallow, and organic duck fats, as well as organic extra virgin oil, and raw organic whole milks, butter, and fats. In short, healthy, good, saturated fats are what the body needs to function. Healthy saturated fats are the preferred fuel for the brain, the heart, the nerves, and the immune system. If you need to learn more about healthy good fats, please read Mary G. Enig's book entitled: *Know your Fats: The Complete Primer for Understanding the Nutrition of Fats, Oils and Cholesterol.*

3. PROPERLY PREPARED NUTRIENT-DENSE WHOLE FOODS

Two-thirds of an adult diet should ideally be raw, organic fresh, green, leafy vegetables to keep the food enzymes live. Live food contains live enzymes. These are the body's real workers that rebuild and regenerate all the cells—keeping them healthy and able to fight infections. Live enzymes are very fragile; they easily get killed with poor food preparation practices such as overcooking, microwaving, or over-processing. The organic pasture-raised macronutrients such as: proteins, fats, and organic and unprocessed carbohydrates, are found mostly in green leafy vegetables. The body's physiology hasn't evolved much despite the industrialization of agricultural farming and food processing. It still needs primarily simple, fresh, live, organic, properly-prepared, nutrient-dense whole foods.

I give a comprehensive six-hour workshop on this subject every second Saturday of the month in my clinic. The class is called the "Nutritional Bootcamp." If you are interested, please book an appointment by calling 832.463.4526.

4. CUTTING OUT REFINED GRAINS AND SUGARY TREATS

Essentially, the body is not designed to eat refined and processed carbohydrates daily—maybe once a week or at a minimal amount of around 15g per day. I truly believe that the human body is not built to constantly digest refined carbohydrates as its main source of energy. These treats are the most inefficient form of energy source for the body in the long term. Too much energy and insulin are required for the body to convert these carbs to a usable glucose form that the muscles can absorb. These carbs also burn so quickly that your body will require more and more throughout the day. Refined carbohydrates can cause increased inflammation and wreak havoc on your body's systems. To add insult to injury, refined grain foods and sugary treats suppress your immune system approximately three to four hours after digestion. What is not healthy for your overall body health is surely not ideal for your foot health.

5. CAFFEINE AND DEHYDRATION

I need to include the role of caffeine on dehydration because this too has an impact on overall health. Drinking too much caffeine throughout the day, without drinking your required water intake, causes dehydration. Caffeine is a diuretic substance; one cup of a caffeinated drink may take away three or four glasses of fluids from the body. The kidneys use approximately three or four glasses-worth of water just to filter and extract water from a caffeinated or sugary drink.

Over time, chronic dehydration will dry up the soft tissues, joints, and tendons, including the disks in the spine, knees, and shoulders. Chronic dehydration can result from drinking a massive amount of caffeinated drink without drinking enough water. Ideally, you need to drink half of your body weight equal to ounces with a pinch of sea salt in every eight ounces of filtered water (preferably Himalayan sea salt). (For example, a 160-pound male or female should drink 80 ounces of water a day, or ten 8-ounce glasses.)

Chronic unintended dehydration will also affect the adrenal glands, sleep, and the heart. For some people, it increases their heart rate and could cause tachycardia. For some women, the caffeine weakens their bladder muscles. If you need to read more about this matter, I strongly suggest reading the book *Water* by Dr. Batmanghelidj, MD. This book is required reading for all patients in my clinic.

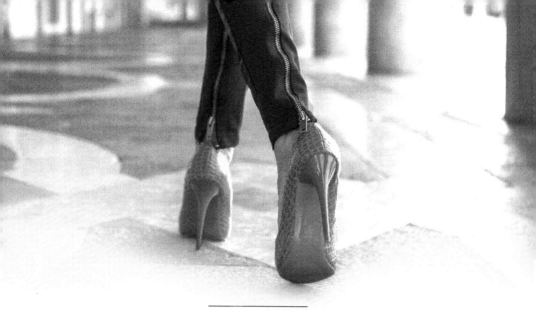

CHAPTER 11

Caring for Your Legs and Feet

"Most people have no idea how good their body is designed to feel."

—KEVIN TRUDEAU

Believe it or not, more people take better care of their car than they do of their health, especially of their legs and feet. Your legs and feet slave away all day long, especially if you are walking in high-heeled shoes daily. They deserve to be cared for with love and tenderness. This chapter discusses necessary maintenance routines for the feet and legs. These are simple but practical suggestions that will help to ensure healthy legs and feet.

1. GET PEDICURES REGULARLY

Maintain a regular pedicure habit at home or professionally, at least once every three weeks. If you decide to do it outside your home, make sure to check for proper hygiene practices in any nail salon to prevent fungal or bacterial contamination to your feet. Be sure to trim your toenails properly in straight cuts to avoid ingrown toenails.

2. DAILY LEG AND FOOT WASH

While in the shower, use foot scrub and a washcloth to exfoliate the dead skin on your legs and feet. A daily leg and foot wash will also stimulate the lymphatic system of the legs and feet. The lymphatic system has a significant role in the immune system, especially regarding the feet. Use mild organic soap on your skin only every other day. Daily use of soap is not necessary, because it will dry out your skin and remove the good bacteria from the skin's surface.

3. USE ORGANIC SKIN LOTION

After your shower, always apply organic skin lotion to restore moisture and rehydrate your skin. The use of organic skin lotion will prevent dryness and skin breakouts. It makes the skin soft and tight. I usually use organic extra virgin coconut oil on my skin daily. If you cannot read and spell the ingredients listed on the lotion label, do not put it on your skin. They are more likely to be toxic chemicals that will poison and attack your body. Also, if the ingredients are not edible, please do not put it on your skin. Your skin pores are like micro-mouths all over your body that will directly absorb ingredients into your blood stream. The lotion therefore has direct access to your bloodstream and your immune system, with little protection from your skin barrier of good bacteria.

4. SOAK YOUR FEET WEEKLY

Two standard foot-soaking methods are very doable at home at a meager cost. I advise making these a weekly or monthly routine to maintain health and prevent diseases.

It is very beneficial for feet to soak with Epsom salts for at least one hour at a time. Soaking will draw out accumulated blood toxins through the pores of the feet, and replenish the needed magnesium back into the feet. This soak is also good for relaxing feet muscles. Another good soak for the feet is a mix of organic extra virgin coconut oil with raw coconut vinegar, in a one-to-one ratio. This soak is very effective with any fungal infection and, at the same time, detoxifies your blood. The extra virgin coconut oil has an antimicrobial property and kills any harmful microbes, whether fungus, bacteria, or virus. The amazing thing is that the organic extra virgin coconut oil will NOT kill the good bacteria in the body.

I had a patient who had had a foot fungus for over twenty years. She used to see her podiatrist monthly for her persistent fungal infection. It went away and was resolved completely after a few weeks of soaking daily for one hour with the organic extra virgin coconut oil and coconut vinegar concoction.

5. SPRAY YOUR FEET WITH ANTIPERSPIRANT.

If your feet tend to be sweaty, there is a possibility that you have a vitamin D_3 deficiency, along with other mineral deficiencies. Until you correct these deficiencies, you could spray between your toes with antiperspirant to minimize sweating. This will also control foot odor.

6. ELEVATE YOUR FEET DAILY

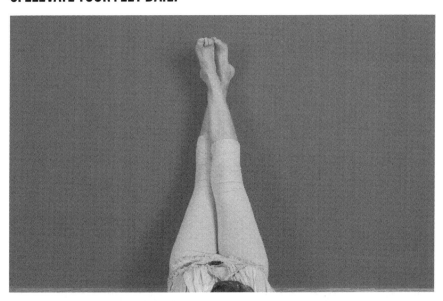

Fig. 41. *Elevating Both Legs on the Wall for 15 minutes to 20 minutes*

Elevate your feet at least twelve inches higher than your heart for fifteen to twenty minutes, no more, no less. I usually prop up my feet on my bed headboard while listening to music or praying my nightly Rosary. Elevating your legs is the most efficient way of helping the tired blood from your feet return to your heart for blood re-oxygenation and rejuvenation. Recovery for your tired feet and legs will be much faster this way and they will be ready for the next day. It also prevents varicose veins and reduces swelling in the feet.

Always use a timer when doing this exercise, because more than twenty minutes is not good for you either. It will drain away too much of the feet's blood circulation. This can cause foot pain due to excessive blood emptying.

No amount of leg stocking support will equal the benefits of gravity-assisted leg circulation emptying. I have never missed doing this daily for the last thirty years since I started wearing high-heeled shoes. My legs and feet feel so much better after elevation. I also feel less tired and ready for the next day.

7. WEEKLY FOOT MASSAGE

I recommend getting weekly massages, since we use our feet so much daily. Massage is good for the feet and stimulates the immune system. Massage is almost like taking one thousand doses of vitamins, whether the massage is for the feet or the entire body.

8. DAILY FOOT EXERCISES

Since I wear high heels at work daily, I routinely do feet elevation with foot exercises and stretches at night. The foot exercise called "sole energizer" is a good foot maintenance routine. For detailed foot exercises instructions, please visit www.holisticptclinic.com.

9. EARTHING

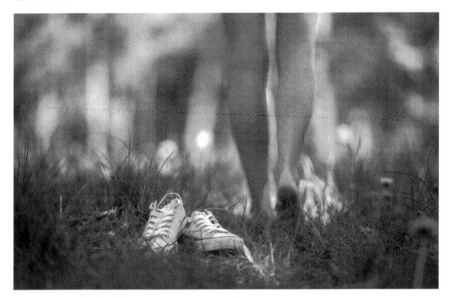

Fig. 42. *Grounding or Earthing–Barefoot Walking on Grass[1]*

Your body is electrically and magnetically charged. It maintains a healthy balance of positive and negative electrons for optimal health. The positive electrons increase when the body is experiencing inflammation. The negative electrons are the good guys; they neutralize and repair the inflammatory positive electrons. Fortunately, there is a free unlimited source of healthy negative electrons ... Mother Earth! She is the best source of the anti-inflammatory negative electrons. It is believed that Mother Earth gets its negative electrons during thunderstorms and lightning strikes. Every time a lightning bolt hits the ground, she is recharged. We call this Earthing ...

Earthing means walking barefoot on a beach, on a dew-moistened grass, on concrete, or on a tile floor and receiving the best direct access to Mother Earth's negative electrons. Mother Earth supplies us with gentle energy, perhaps as Vitamin G (G for ground energy). When we make direct contact with the surface of the earth, our bodies receive an infusion of gentle energy that makes us feel better, fast.

As life happens throughout the day, the negative anti-inflammatory electrons get used up, and positive electrons become dominant. Eventually, fatigue occurs, and inflammatory processes set in. There are two ways to access Vitamin G.

First, walking barefoot on a beach, grass, concrete, or tile floor, gives anti-inflammatory negative electrons recharged back to your body by reentering through the soles of your feet. Exposing your bare feet to the ground regenerates the nerves in your feet thus reenergizing your whole body and its internal organs. It is also the best natural blood thinner without pharmaceutical drugs. It is not a good idea to do Earthing if you are taking a blood thinner. Ideally, you are supposed to wait between one-to-two weeks after weaning off a blood thinner before you can do Earthing.

The moment I get home from work, I take off my shoes and walk barefoot on my tile floor while working in my kitchen. This restores my calf muscles and lets my bare feet ground to the earth, adding anti-inflammatory electrons to recharge my body at the end of the day.

I strongly suggest plantar fasciitis sufferers walk barefoot on the ground as much as they can tolerate. It is the best anti-inflammatory antidote for a swollen fascia of the foot and for the rest of the body.

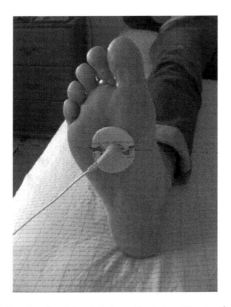

Fig. 43. *Earthing Patch on the Sole of the Foot*[2]

The second way to increase negative electrons is by grounding at night indoors. You can recharge your body with negative electrons while you sleep. There is a gadget that I highly recommend called a grounding kit, designed by an electrician, Clinton Ober, with Dr. Stephen Sinatra, MD. It is a simple device that connects you to the ground outlet—the third eye on the electrical wall outlet. It comes as a basic Earthing patch kit, grounding bed sheets, pillow cases, computer bands, and foot and car pads. With a minimal investment, it is worth trying because it has so many health benefits.

I use the grounding kit at night to access more negative electrons while sleeping. It energizes and helps the body improve blood flow and prevents and reverses the Rouleaux phenomena (red blood cells sticking together creating slowed circulation).

There are reliable scientific research studies showing that grounding at night will help with sleep apnea. I have hundreds of patients benefitting from this grounding principle. Think of it this way, if it does not work, it is a small investment of money (approximately $70 to $300 depending on which Earthing products you use).

If you are interested in learning more about Earthing, I strongly suggest you check out Dr. Stephen Sinatra, MD, or visit www.earthing.com. Dr. Sinatra is a cardiologist who pioneered scientific studies about Earthing. Also, look on www.mercola.com for more articles and featured studies on Earthing.

Chapter Notes

1. http://www.natures-blessings.org/feetGrounding.jpg
2. http://thenaturalmedicalhealthwell.com/wp-content/uploads/2012/08/EARTHING-Patch-on-Kidney-1.jpg

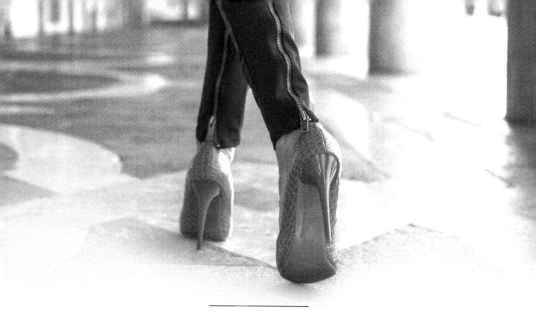

CHAPTER 12

TLC for Your Shoes

"Good shoes takes you good places."

T his is the last chapter but it is nevertheless very important. Buying and wearing a nice pair of high heels is just the beginning. The biggest mistake that most high heel wearers make is neglecting to care for their shoes after bringing them home. Giving the proper TLC to your high-heeled shoes will protect your investment by keeping them looking better longer. Every style of high-heeled shoe requires special attention after you wear them. With these tips, your high-heeled shoes may outlast you...

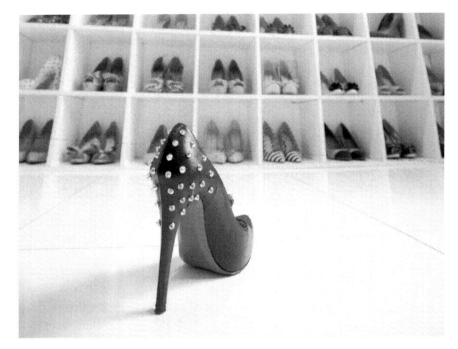

Fig. 44. *Shoe Organizer*

1. COAT NEW HIGH-HEELED SHOES WITH A WATERPROOF PROTECTOR SPRAY.

It will keep the shoe surface from getting deformed and marred if they do get wet from water or rain. There are different brand names available; most of them do the job.

2. ALTERNATE PAIRS.

Alternating different pairs of shoes is suitable not only for variety but also it is good for the shoe. This way your shoes will not be worn out in a short period of time. Your shoes will have time to rest and breathe in between wearing, and any residual moisture can dry out.

3. CLEAN THE INSIDES.

Cleaning the inside of your shoes is of particular importance to prevent or remove shoe odor. Swab them with alcohol or a drop of tea tree oil, an antifungal agent. Be sure not to splash the fluid to avoid staining the leather.

4. CLEAN THE SOLES OF YOUR HIGH-HEELED SHOES BEFORE STORING.

Cleaning the shoe soles before storing is a good routine to develop. Any dirt and debris could also ruin the soles of your shoes when stored for an extended period. Your shoes are the number one culprit in bringing dirt into your house, and that is why it is a good idea to clean shoes before bringing them inside.

5. ALWAYS STORE YOUR HIGH-HEELED SHOES IN THEIR PROPER SHOE BOXES.

Keep your high heels in their original shoe box with corresponding picture and/or labels outside the shoe box for easy organization of your closet. You can stack the shoe boxes efficiently without deforming their shape. Although, if you have special display shelves for your high-heeled shoes, you do not need to use boxes.

6. CONSIDER ADDING TAPS AND HALF-SOLES OF RUBBER TO THE BOTTOMS.

Taps and half-soles are high-heeled shoe reinforcements that will protect and add many years to the life of your shoes. You may need to bring your shoes to a good shoe repair shop to get someone to install them for you.

7. ORGANIZE FOR SEASON AND COLOR.

It is easier to put together an outfit when your high-heeled shoes are organized by season, and by color. Rather than looking through every box to find a pair that matches your outfit, save yourself some time with an organized shoe closet. Besides, it gives such pleasure and satisfaction every morning when everything is laid out and organized.

8. LEATHER CARE

Take time to do your leather care at the end of every season to maintain your high-heeled shoes properly. Recondition the leather if necessary. Your favorite high-heeled shoes will last longer and maintain their shape and integrity with proper leather care.

9. SHOESHINE

Invest in a routine shoeshine or polish for high-heeled shoes as needed. It is imperative to have clean shoes on high heels because a poorly maintained high-heeled shoe makes a bad first impression. Besides, high heels will not last very long if they are badly maintained.

10. SHOE FORMS

Always use shoe forms or paper to stuff your shoes, in order to maintain their original shape. Always place your high-heeled shoes in proper shoe storage for the next season or until the next time you use them.

11. WORN OUT HEELS

Replace worn out heels to maintain shoe integrity and safety. Worn out heels give a negative first impression, not to mention that they will slowly ruin the main structural heel of your shoes. Knowing a good cobbler helps.

12. GIVE AWAY

Donate to charity or to a good cause to unload your closet. Try to give a pair of shoes away every time you buy a new one. There is always another woman out there who can use your unused pair of lovely high-heeled shoes. Share the love ... the love of shoes!

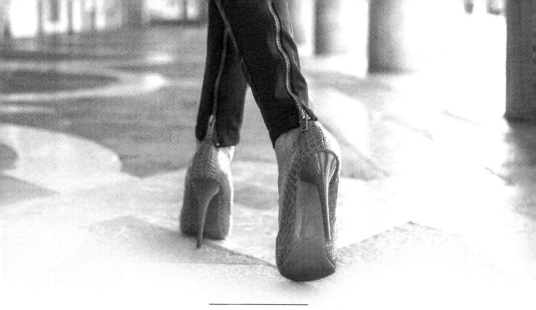

The reason why I wrote this book...

Throughout the ages high heels have been used by nobility and royalty as a sign of their superiority over their subjects. Similarly, today women can wear a pair of heels to her social advantage. Yet there are many misconceptions about high heels. They have been blamed for most foot maladies from bunions to neuroma, and ankle injuries. That is like blaming a car for injuring and killing people in an accident. Let's not forget a minor detail: it is the operator's skill level that is usually at fault, not the car.

We have learned that high heels can be good for you! They are good for your brain: proper posture with proper standing dynamic balance while walking on high heels improves brain function. High heels also boost one's attractiveness to the opposite sex. High heel walking is a good exercise for strengthening your core muscles, pelvic floor muscles, and leg muscles. It helps to get good professional and quick social response from men. It also helps give good first impressions. Finally, high heels improve one's psyche and sex appeal with grace and confidence.

The sexy art of high heel walking is a unique skill set. To be sexy, confident, and pain-free on high heels, one has to master this particular skill. High heel walking is a learned skill, not an instinctual one. Learning the skill on your own without instruction is not ideal in order to be able to do it correctly, safely, and without injury. The majority of women who try to figure out high heel walking on their own usually experience foot pain, suffering... and HUMILIATION! However, these outcomes don't stop most women from buying high heels without learning the proper High heel walking technique. It is very beneficial to learn the whole process: starting with how to shoe shop, choosing the proper shoe fit, learning the proper posture barefoot and with the high heels, then learning the proper high heel walk, the aftercare of your feet, good body and foot nutrition, the proper shoe storage, and proper shoe care. This way you will be able to achieve the sexy high heel walk with grace and confidence, safely, pain-free, and without injury. A perfect reason to enjoy and cherish many, many, many, more high-heeled shoes to come!

"You can never take too much care over the choice of your shoes. Too many women think that they are unimportant, but the real proof of an elegant woman is what is on her feet."

—CHRISTIAN DIOR